I0115926

Published by Robert Boyce

http://www.robboycefitness.com
Phone: 414-861-0879

First Edition

ISBN - 978-0-578-15838-9

Book Design by Stone Hedge Graphics, Inc.

Printed in the United States of America

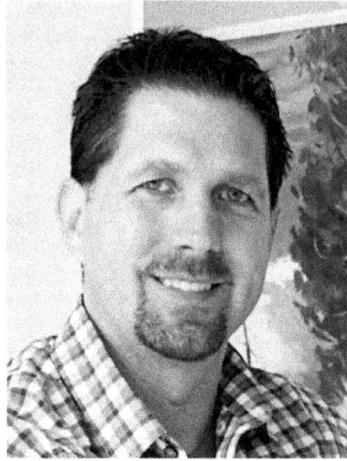

Robert Boyce BS, CSCS

Fitness Transformation Specialist

Hi. I'm Rob. As a certified personal trainer, I have been helping women transform their bodies for the last 15 years. One thing I have learned is that whether your 20 or 40 the formula for changing your body doesn't change. Don't be fooled by all the quick fix diets out there. With all the hype and confusion out there I will show any woman, that regardless of their age or situation, they can have the best body possible. Now don't just take my word for it. You will meet three women from three different decades that overcame adversity and followed the simple principles to get the body they always wanted. You won't just learn the nuts and bolts of how to change your body, because let's be realistic, this information can be looked up in seconds on the Internet. You will be motivated by their stories as well as many others. You will learn from their mistakes as well as their clever ideas to stay on track in a world where women wear many hats in a hectic lifestyle. Hear real stories from real women in real life situations.

Are you ready for the new you?!

How does she do it

Meet your inspiration

Dedicated to:

My mother and father, Bob and Rikki, who have always believed in me. They gave me the opportunity to receive a great education and always supported me in my quest to reach my goals and dreams.

Cheryl whose tough love approach to life inspired me to always keep pushing forward

All the women who have struggled with their bodies and who have tried every quick fix and have failed because of misinformation and lack of a simple plan.

Acknowledgement:

Mary, who listened and applied the simple principles that I taught her. Even though there may have been a struggle or two, she didn't let me down. She stayed accountable not only to her self but also to me. It didn't hurt that I left a seed in her head that if she failed then I would have failed too.

Christina, who beat the odds by keeping the weight off and made fitness a part of her life

My lady bootcampers: For five years I learned as much from you as you hopefully did from me. Through the days of heat, cold, rain, sleet, snow, tornado type winds and fires, you always showed up ready to make it happen. This list is not all inclusive, however those that are burned in my head forever are: Jody M, Jodi B, Cherie B, Vicki, Sue S, Sue B, Denise I, Anna L, Amy K, Rose S, Janice, Kathy K , Trish, Karen N, Kathryn M.

A few special Clients from Motion Fitness Club who will always be part of my life as they were an inspiration to me early in my career. Faye G, Renee K, Ann T, Kelley K, Mary Beth S, Lawne C.

Introduction

It's finally time to make a change. Not just a simple change but a life-altering change.

It would be easy for me to sit here and tell you what you need to do, but I may not know your story. You may have a busy schedule and limited time to exercise. You may have three or more kids that take up most of your free time. You may not be able to afford a gym membership. You may be thinking there is no way you can lose 30 percent or more of your body weight. You may be a single parent that works several jobs and is always exhausted. You may think it's just not possible to look like you did 20 years ago.

You're probably thinking that it's easy for me to tell you what to do—but your situation is different. How can I help you when I haven't even walked one step in your shoes?

You can put all your questions to rest because you are going to learn how to get results regardless of your situation. You will learn tried-and-tested concepts, techniques, workouts, eating plans, tricks, shortcuts, and much more from women who have been in your shoes. Yes, these women have been in your shoes, and, hopefully, soon you will be following in theirs.

But before we change your life, let me tell you a little bit about my inspiration because, let's face it, being inspired motivates! Motivation gets you started, and habit keeps you going.

My health and fitness voyage started when I was finishing high school. I was always active, playing sports, working out, and getting fit, and I was interested in how the body works and what makes things tick.

My father, who was in his late forties at the time, had to have heart surgery. I was about to enter college and was always interested in computers, so I felt that was the route to go. However, my dad, who had helped me with everything in my life, needed some direction.

He smoked one or two packs of cigarettes each day and, after a long day of work, sat in his recliner with his remote control nearby. By the end of the night, he would have eaten a 5-gallon tub of popcorn, usually with one quarter of it all over his chest or on the floor. The only way popcorn wasn't on the floor is if our dog, Freddy, had licked it off of him or eaten the kernels that fell on the cushions.

I wanted to help my dad. That's the least I could do since he and my mother, my biggest cheerleader, were paying my college tuition. I am very grateful for my education because, without it, I would not be in a position to help you today.

The internet was in its infancy when I was in college, and it wasn't easy to get good information about health and fitness. My first assignment in a management information systems class was to find out what was on David Letterman that evening. It wasn't as simple as it is today. It took me 10 minutes to complete the task; today it would take 10 seconds.

The professor told us that soon we would be able to order flowers online or even book an airline flight. We all thought he was crazy. Little did we know that his predictions were spot on.

Unfortunately, over the past 20 years, the internet has gone crazy. My last Google search found more than a billion results for books on fitness and 136 million results for books on changing your body. An Amazon search brought up a thousand books on body transformation, 227,000 books on fitness, and more than 65,000 books on nutrition. So, I'm not sure which is worse: not having any information or having too much information.

You can find any answer you want on how to change your body. The problem is that a lot of the information is contradictory, which is one of the reasons I'm here to set you straight. I want to make fitness relatable to every woman in the simplest, most non-intimidating way.

My post-college career in fitness started in a hospital wellness setting, where patients' insurance companies offered incentives to get fit and do things to help prevent disease. Not only did I learn some great tests, procedures, and consulting techniques, but my eyes were opened up pretty darn wide that medicine is a business. I didn't see a lot of compassion toward helping people. I'm not saying that it doesn't happen, but I knew that if I wanted to help people, it wasn't going to be in that setting.

When you start your journey to transform your body once and for all, there is one thing you need to keep in mind: There is a difference between getting healthy (keeping sickness and disease away) and transforming your body into being sculpted like a Greek goddess. Don't get me wrong, you can have both, but they don't always go hand in hand. My first boss was a vegetarian, so you might think that because he ate healthy and didn't eat any bad stuff he would have had a great-looking body, right? Well, the truth was that he looked like he ate fast food and never worked out. This is just an example that eating healthy doesn't guarantee a great, or even good-looking, body.

I have worked with thousands of women, and getting results doesn't change too much regardless of age. I have also heard just about every excuse as to why a woman can't workout or achieve the body she wants, and, oh my goodness, there are some doozies! "I just like to eat rich foods." "I'm too old." "I have to stop working out because I have sweat in my eyes." "I just don't have time." And the most recent one I heard when a lady was looking to cancel her fitness membership at the club I now manage was that she didn't need to work out in summer because she got her cardiovascular activity from sky diving.

Maybe I am missing something here, but we can apparently justify any excuse.

The truth is that women make excuses when they're not ready, when they feel they don't have what it takes to succeed, or when they have truly tried but just didn't have the correct information and consider themselves a failure.

The good news is, if you were following a program and didn't get the results you were looking for, you didn't fail. Your program failed you.

There are too many women who give up without realizing that whatever program they were on was flawed from the beginning. It wasn't their fault, yet they blame themselves. It didn't give them the tools they need to succeed in the long term.

I'm not here to battle with scientists about what foods can be harmful to you or which ones can fight disease. I'm here to put the end to the word "diet" and show you how simple, not easy, it really is to transform your body at any age.

You won't just hear it from me though. Even though I will give you everything you need to succeed, you'll also see how three special women did it. I'm certain you will be able to relate to one of our not-so-common women whether you're in your 20s, 30s, 40s, or beyond.

These women live the same lives you do and still found a way to look their best. These ladies will inspire you and make you realize that anyone can change their body. You just need to be armed with the right advice, which I will supply, and be committed to follow the plan.

Chapter 1:   Ambushed by misinformation

I will take out all the sugar coating and give it to you straight, whether you want to hear it or not. As many of my clients will tell you, I don't baby them and let them think it is ok to fall off the wagon and give up. Why would I? That would just give them false hope, which is what most of those quick-fix diets do already. They have most people brainwashed with tricky marketing and hype.

People then blame themselves for failing a program that was dead from the start.

The other day, I picked up a few items from the grocery store, and I strolled by the book aisle. I like to stay on top of the next "best-kept secret" in the diet world. Guess what? I was not disappointed.

I came across four must-have books (I'm being sarcastic here): the 8-hour diet, the 17-day diet, the digest diet, and the fast diet. While skimming through them, at least one was backed by journal studies, but I know how these studies can be manipulated. They all had magic ingredients to change your body. It was kind of a comic relief for me, but, boy, how confusing to most people, especially if you really need help.

The funny thing is that they were all so different but were going to deliver the same results. Some were even written by doctors. Did you know that most doctors take only a single nutrition course in medical school? Yet I think when some people see the title "doctor" preceding the author's name, they assume the book must be worthwhile and credible.

Even Dr. Phil has a fitness/weight-loss book, and I don't recall him having any fitness background. I bet if Dr. Seuss wrote a fitness book, it would be a best seller! There is a little phrase I remember from a "Brady Bunch" episode when Greg was going to buy a car from a friend. The car didn't run very well, but his buddy said that it only needed a few tweaks from a screwdriver to make it purr like a kitten. The phrase was "caveat emptor," which translates to "buyer beware." Just because you see the word "doctor" by an author's name, it doesn't mean the book is the holy grail of fitness.

Additionally, when you see research cited from an academic journal, be wary. It's funny how certain things can get left out of an article or the article can be taken out of context, which can make the results look misleading. You can find research out there to back up any idea or concept. Testimonials and results from real people speak volumes, not mumbo jumbo designed to mislead you and make you fail or a supermodel saying this is what she did to get in shape when, in reality, she is a paid spokesperson.

Before you learn what the plan is, it is important to understand some of the reasons you may have failed in the past. Most people blame themselves for their fitness failures, but it really isn't their fault. How can you succeed if you think you are getting information from trusted sources but, in reality, it is misinformation?

I have worked alongside some great personal trainers throughout my career. One trainer, Stephanie, was asked by a big-name company to represent one of their fat-melting supplements. She was pregnant at the time, and they asked her to come out and take some pictures immediately following her child's birth. Then, they gave her some time to get back into competition form and arranged for a second photo shoot. The finished commercial suggested that sometimes life gets in the way, but this product had helped her lose 31 pounds. Funny that it didn't mention being pregnant was what got in the way!

Yes, it was very deceiving, but did you know that the testimonials are what sell these products? I'm sure many of you have seen these commercials, and this product in particular, only to run to the store to purchase them thinking you found the magic bullet. Can supplements aid you in your quest for the perfect body? Sure they can, but remember they are a supplement and, by definition, something that completes or enhances something else.

A supplement by itself is not going to get you the body you want. If anyone tells you that their supplement is the magic pill, just laugh and walk away because the magic pill doesn't exist.

Chapter 2:   **Consumer beware**

Who can you trust these days? Even big food companies are pulling the wool over your eyes. Do you use nonfat cooking spray? If you look at the label, it says "for fat-free cooking," but if you look at the ingredients, which are listed from most to least, it starts with olive oil or canola oil or some type of oil. Oil is fat.

So how do they get away with saying it is fat-free? The FDA says if a serving size is less than .5 grams, then companies can say it is fat-free when, in reality, it is essentially 100% fat.

Some of those labels are actually comical. They say a serving size is one-third of a second. Come on, who can take their finger off the nozzle in that amount of time? That would have to be a world record. And, even if you could take your finger off in time, it is still fat.

In addition to fooling you, they are also quite possibly hurting you.

Have you heard of high-fructose corn syrup? According to all the food companies, it's no different than sugar. But now Yoplait's newest commercial is telling the whole world that we should be happy because they are taking high-fructose corn syrup out of *some* of their yogurts. Why take it out if it's harmless and no different than sugar? It still has 26 grams of sugar even though it is 99% fat free.

Fat free, sugar free, high carb, low carb—what do I do?

Did you hear the latest from Gatorade? They had a chemical in their drinks that is also found in flame retardants; according to Pepsi spokeswoman Molly Cater, it has been removed.

Even Subway was recently under scrutiny for having an unfamiliar and hard-to-pronounce chemical in its bread called azodicarbonamide. Subway says it's an extremely common bread ingredient that helps strengthen dough. This ingredient is banned in Europe and Australia. Did I mention this ingredient is also used in yoga mats and shoe soles to add elasticity? This ingredient has also been recently removed from the bread-ingredient list at Subway but is still in many other fast-food-chain products.

How about all the infomercial gadgets guaranteeing you a flat stomach and six-pack abs? Remember the really obnoxious guy with the long blonde hair? He was quite the character and has actually resurfaced again. I'm sure everyone has at least one of these products in their basement being used as a clothes hanger or stuffed under a bed collecting dust.

Some of these gadgets might give you a strong midsection or help you burn some calories, but no gadget in the world is going to single handedly remove the fat sitting so nicely on top of those abs. That's why you will usually see a disclaimer at the bottom saying "results not typical" while the fitness model makes it look so simple. Abs are made in the kitchen; it takes healthy eating and an exercise plan to remove the fat, not a single gadget.

Even your treadmill, stationary bike, elliptical, and watches that figure out how many calories you have burned can be misleading. Most of these cardio devices overestimate your calorie burn, some by as much as 42 percent. In their defense, figuring out the science of calories in not that simple. So use the units as a guideline, not an absolute number.

5

If you are going to try and get a ballpark figure, you must enter your weight into the machine or it will assume you are a 150-pound male. If you are really curious, an intense workout will burn about 100 calories every ten minutes.

Got milk? Who drinks skim, 1%, 2%? Do you thing that 1% milk is one-percent fat? It's not! Skim milk is actually fat free, however, 1% milk is actually 17% fat. Two percent is 36% fat, and whole milk is 50% fat.

How do they get away with that you ask? They do it by weight, not the actual calories. Picture a gallon of milk. It is 99% water and only 1 percent of the rest. So, by weight, it is 1% fat. When you look at the actual calories you are consuming, the percent of fat is much higher depending on what type you are drinking. I don't typically put milk on my list of clean foods because it has a lot of sugar and has inflammatory properties, but that topic is for another book on health not body transformation.

We all love to read the latest fitness magazines so we know which supplements to buy and what the best exercises are to mold a great tush, right? Did you know that most of these magazines are owned by supplement companies? It's no wonder that the fit people in those magazines say they use the products that are conveniently advertised there. The magazines are just a vehicle to sell their products. This is just another little magic act played at the consumers' expense.

Gluten free is the latest craze. Many people who don't have celiac disease are buying these products simply because they make them feel better. Sales in 2013 topped an estimated 4 billion dollars. The bad news is that labeling for gluten-free products was not regulated until August 2014. What does that mean? Deceitful food companies could label anything "gluten free." Now, all gluten-free products must contain less than 20 parts per million of gluten.

You need to be aware of the untruths and deceits around you. You really can't go wrong when transforming your body if you stick to the basics of clean eating and moderate exercise. Look at the chiseled Greek statues from hundreds of years ago. Do you think they used any secret pills? The rest is just hype, and these marketers get paid a lot of money for you to believe them.

Chapter 3:   **What has all this food done to us?**

Take a look around and see what is happening: Obesity is an epidemic.

I read a study that says adult obesity rates could exceed 60% in thirteen states by 2030. If obesity rates continue at this pace, the number of type 2 diabetes, heart disease, and strokes could increase 10 times between now and 2020 and double again by 2030. It seems like statistics don't really scare people because most people think that it won't happen to them.

What's even scarier is that, according to the Centers for Disease Control and Prevention, 16.9% of children and adolescents ages 2 to 19 are obese. Since 1980, childhood obesity has almost tripled.

Dr. Kenneth Cooper, the godfather of aerobic training, has said, "Along with the increase in childhood obesity we're beginning to see an epidemic of adult onset, or type 2, diabetes in children 9 to 12. If that child develops diabetes before they're 14 years of age they are shortening their life span by 17 to 27 years. This has reached such a state that this may be the first generation in which the parents outlive the children."

I think part of the problem is that we as consumers get upset if we don't get our money's worth when we go out to eat. We expect a great big plate of food pouring over the sides. Portion control to most people is an afterthought when they're unbuttoning their pants after a gluttonous experience.

Chapter 4:   **You have to be ready, not "kinda" ready**

Some of you have never had the feeling of being in great shape and have only thought about having the body of your dreams. Others have experienced what feeling and looking good is all about. It really doesn't matter if you have been there before or not, because, as your life changes, so does your lifestyle. We all need some guidance when we enter a new phase of life.

So many women look to change their bodies for the wrong reasons. If you aren't doing it for yourself, you might as well stop reading and come back when you are ready. That word "ready" has really hit home with me lately. I took on a new client and asked her if she was ready. She said she was ready, so I dug in and gave it my all. I prepared food plans, workouts and a comprehensive plan of what it was going to take to reach this lady's goal. A few weeks into the program, the excuses started popping out like fish out of a barrel.

She told me that I didn't understand because she had a husband and kids and worked two hours per day during the school year. Well, this sounds like the life of almost every woman over 35. Actually, it sounds much easier than what most women I help battle on a daily basis.

What did I not understand? We all have situations, and I have a hard time listening to excuses. She is no longer in my program. If you are making excuses, you are not ready, it's that simple. I believe you have to clear some things off your plate and open up some space for yourself to truly commit and be ready for a change. Am I saying you should be selfish? Yes, I am.

9

I recently had the chance to meet David and Rebecca Nielsen. They were on ABC's "Extreme Makeover" weight-loss edition 2013. David told me that not everyone on the show makes it to the TV screen because some people just aren't "ready."

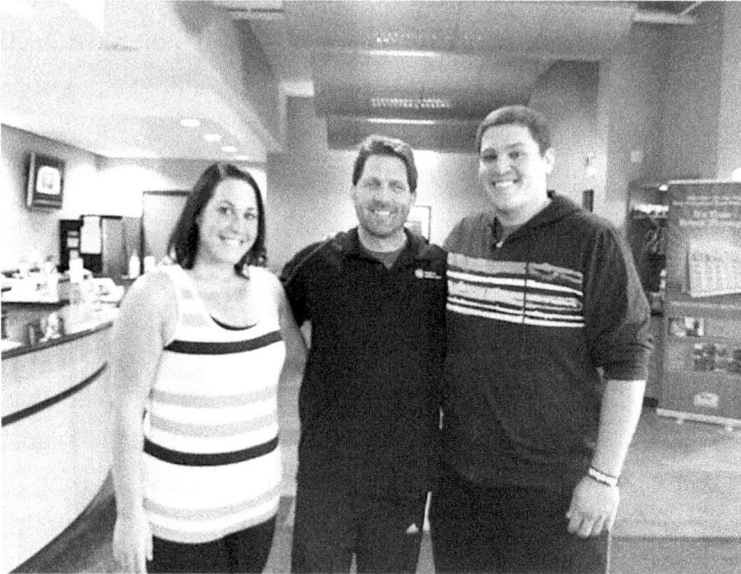

Meeting David and Rebecca Nielsen from ABC's "Extreme Makeover" weight-loss edition 2013

He lost half of his bodyweight, more than 200 pounds. When I asked him what kept him going, he said it was his short-term success. The first week, he lost 18 pounds, and the second week he lost 17 pounds. After his short-term success, he told himself that he was not ever turning back. While discussing both David and Becca's success, I told Rebecca that only 1 in 6 people that lose a significant amount of weight will keep it off. She said she was going to change those odds. After diving in deeper to look at the success of this brother-sister team, I was disturbed to hear that the final month of weight loss consisted of diuretics, laxatives, and body cleanses. This really doesn't teach people how to survive in the real world, when the show ends and it's back to business as usual, which is why so many people gain the weight back after these Hollywood-type programs.

You can't make a life-altering transformation because someone wants you to or told you to. In the Nielsons' case, their father kept telling them they needed to lose weight. He even bought them a home gym, which they never used.

You have to do it for you, and you have to be ready for the challenge. I often run weight-loss and body-fat-loss challenges in my boot camps, and some ladies just aren't ready, whatever the reason may be. I can't change that. I can try to motivate and inspire, but, for real success, you need to dig deep and really want it.

Although it's never too late to change your body, that doesn't mean you should put it off forever. Why not be a role model for your family or friends and show them by doing, lead them all down the right path? Maybe you will become someone else's inspiration. How great would that be? Don't forget that you only get one body, and you can't trade it in for a different model.

Chapter 5:   Excuses don't get results

Have you made any excuses over the course of your life as to why you can't change your body and look the way you really desire?

I don't have time	I don't feel like it
My back hurts	I'm too tired
I can't work out, I'm on crutches	I'm too busy
My kids take up my time	Exercise is boring
My husband didn't set the alarm clock	I don't have the motivation
My alarm didn't go off this morning	I'm too old to start a program
I can't afford to go to a gym	I don't have any equipment
I don't know what to do	My dog ate my workout clothes (it worked for homework!)

"Nobody is impressed with how good your excuses are"

I read a funny cartoon: A doctor was talking to a patient and said, "What fits into your busy schedule better, exercising one hour a day or being dead 24 hours a day?" I thought this hit the nail on the head.

You can either pay for exercise now with sweat and hard work or you can pay for disease later. Although this book is about changing your body, not dealing with disease, excuses come in all shapes and sizes and pertain to anything in life. You either want it or you don't. If you want it, you will do whatever it takes to get it.

One morning I was heading to the local high school to teach my women-only boot camp at 5:15 a.m. When I pulled up to the school, lights were flashing, and sirens were sounding. It looked like the circus was coming to town. We walked into the building and had to cover our ears because the fire alarm was going off. I thought it was probably just a test and that the sirens would turn off within a few minutes.

Everyone was excited because we had a weight-loss challenge going on during this session. We got the weigh-ins done, but then the custodian told us there was actually a fire somewhere and we had to leave. I guess the smell of burned rubber should have given it away, but, hey, it was 5 in the morning.

You might think that, in this instance, class was over before it even started because we had no place to workout. However, that was not the case. It was a cold, rainy morning in March, and, in Wisconsin, you just never know what the weather will be like. We aren't cleared for summer weather from Mother Nature until at least June. One of our veteran campers, Cherie, said, "Let's workout outside." I said, "It's raining out." She replied, "So what? We workout in the rain in the summer time."

The next thing you know, everyone was in the parking lot working out. Not one person complained or went home. We could have easily called it a day, but we didn't. Instead of looking for an excuse to leave, they found a solution to workout. It was pretty amazing.

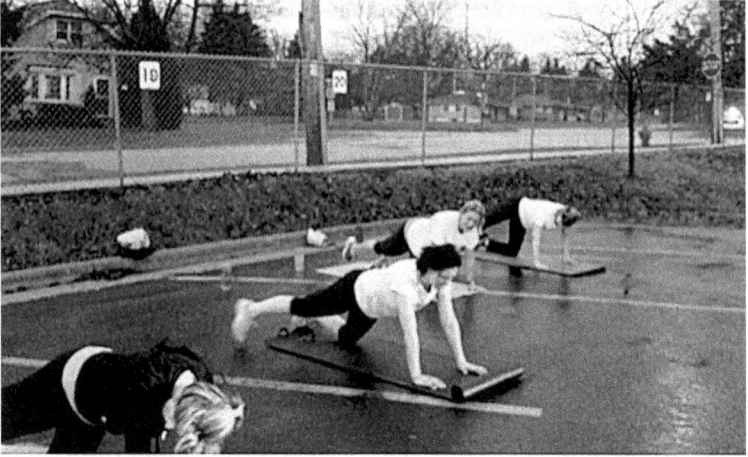

This morning boot camp workout was an amazing example of dedication.

The fire trucks and police cars eventually rolled up to attend to the fire while we finished our workout. This event made the evening news, and school was cancelled for the day in Waterford, Wisconsin. The funny thing was that, with all the commotion going on, no one told us to leave, even though the roads were being blocked off and three different fire departments showed up. The ladies were admiring the firemen, but they still kept moving.

We live in a busy and hectic world, and it's not uncommon for women to work 50 or more hours per week, then put on their taxicab hats and drive their kids to one of many activities, cook dinner, do laundry, help with homework, clean the house, et cetera. It could be very easy to justify why you just can't workout. Don't do it!

Chapter 6: Find a way, not an excuse

I was talking to a client who had taken a break from my women's training class and was going to try to change her body on her own. Vicki noted that she wasn't making excuses, but life had gotten in the way. She could have left it at that, even though her job may have been in jeopardy and she was working 70 hours per week, but she didn't. She told me she was coming back to me for motivation and accountability and was going to reach the goals that she had set for herself. You always have a choice. Sometimes, there are reasons you have to alter your body-transformation goals, but quitting isn't one of them.

This is why accountability is so important: A coach or a good friend isn't going to accept your excuses or reasons for not being successful.

Think about a time when you may have started an exercise program. Initially, you are excited to get up at 5 a.m. and get the ball rolling. (Well, maybe not excited about the getting up at 5 a.m. part.) Three weeks down the road, the alarm goes off, and hitting the snooze button starts to be pretty popular. The next thing you know, you are sleeping in, and, before you know it, you forgot you were even on an exercise program. If you had a partner or coach, this wouldn't happen; someone would be calling you out on your new sleeping transformation.

Just the other day, I called five women that felt like sleeping in rather than coming to class. It was a Friday. Isn't that coincidental? They certainly were not happy with me that morning. As a matter of fact, one of them hung up on me. Nonetheless, I was in their heads, and they definitely thought twice the next time they didn't feel like putting in the effort to come to class. Not only were they accountable to me but also to the rest of the group. Accountability makes sure you are up when you were tired, and, if you had a training partner, you would do the same for them.

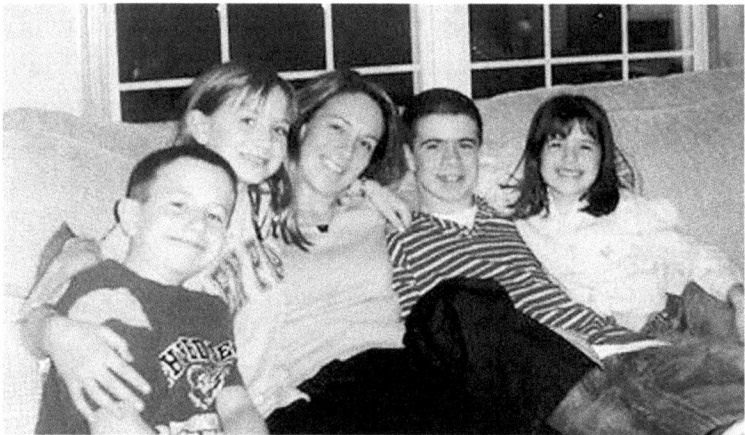

Ann and her children

Meet Ann, a friend and client from several years ago. Ann had a low-back problem that was causing her foot to drop when she walked. This was a serious situation. At the time, she was in her late 30s or early 40s and in great shape; she could have passed for 30. She tried an experimental surgery in 2003 to cure, or at least help, her situation.

She is another example of someone who could have given up and said, since I can't walk, I might as well just take up watching daytime TV. As you may have guessed, that's not what happened. She hired me to train her while recovering.

The workouts were designed with Ann on crutches.

I don't know how many of you have ever simply walked on crutches, but it is not easy. And now we were going to put a safe workout together while on crutches. This was a challenge for both of us and made both of us better people. I designed a program she could do while she was recovering. Ten years later, she is still working out and still looks as good as ever. Just think how her life would be if she had hung up her gym shoes and called it quits. Quitting was not an option.

I asked Ann if I could get a picture of her when she had her crutches for this book and this is what she told me:

That is so funny... I have been thinking about how I want to email you and thank you for all the help you gave me during that terrible time…..I have told the story of me sitting on a leg machine with tears rolling down my face (trying to hide them from you) because it was so hard and I was so sad...but thanks to YOU I did it and made it through all that, so THANK YOU for all the help to keep me going (can you believe it will be 10 years this December!!!).

It was Ann that made the decision to keep going, I just gave her some motivation and a path to follow.

Does you back hurt? Are you feeling sorry for yourself because you feel that there is nothing you can do? You can justify just about anything that you don't feel like doing, but where does that get you?

Your back can't afford not to work out. Yet another great client of mine, Kelley, didn't let her disabling back keep her down. Read her story, and realize you can do anything you put your mind and body to.

I was an active, fit, and trim woman of 5'7" and worked as an intensive care nurse in 1993. At that time, as far as I knew, I was in excellent health when I experienced my first herniated spinal disc. This problem is an inherited genetic predisposition that was certainly aggravated by lifting patients. Unfortunately, this eventually required a laminectomy in June of 1993.

Following the surgery, I returned back to a reasonable activity level and was able to return to nursing. Subsequently, four years later, in 1997 a CT scan and spinal X-ray revealed a collapsed intervertebral disc at the level of L4-L5. Interestingly, my mother, a nurse anesthetist, had developed essentially the same intervertebral collapse when she was also in her late 30s.

At this time, I had a spinal fusion with Simmons metallic plates in my spine to stabilize the vertebrae above and below the collapsed space. Recovery was long, difficult, and extremely painful. Because of my slow progress and inability to ambulate actively and exercise, I began to gain a significant amount of weight. I had never been more miserable in my life, and everyone around me felt frustrated because they couldn't help. Deep depression began to set in.

Then in 2001, I was lifting a potted plant and suddenly felt a very sharp, excruciating pain. This radiated into my legs, and I had great difficulty walking again. Repeat medical evaluation confirmed a new problem, revealing that I had another herniated disc below the plates that were placed in 1993. At this point I had to walk with a cane and wasn't far from being placed in a wheelchair.

Fortunately, I sought re-evaluation by a renowned pain specialist, Dr. Gordon Mortenson. Using a combination of spinal epidural injections and a new combination of drugs, I was then able to handle life a little better. In view of my history and his observations, it was suggested that I may be a candidate for a neuro-stimulator, a new, implantable generator that would continuously send electrical impulses through tiny wires in my spine, essentially limiting my pain.

As a result of my back health, I had physically gone from a size 6 to a size 16-18. I felt like I was 80 years old and unhappy, and to look at me would tell you why. My family encouraged me to consult a personal fitness trainer who had experience in helping people with rehabilitating back problems. I felt I could not do this when I could hardly walk. But I searched out one anyhow, mainly to shut my family up!

On October 20, 2003, I met with personal trainer Rob Boyce. Rob watched me slowly negotiate the staircase and intently observed my condition. I can imagine he felt that this client was a NO-WIN situation, or at least a very tough challenge. However, with Rob's expertise, careful supervision, and encouragement, he created a plan consisting of just the right amount of cardiovascular activity, an overall progressive weight-training program with an emphasis on my back health, and a sound nutrition plan based on my individual body type. He has helped me trim my body, increase my strength, and markedly improve my attitude and motivation.

My husband, a physician, says no one could've believed the dramatic progress that I have made and continue to make. My neuro-stimulato, which at one time was on 24 hours a day, has recently only been on a few times. At this time, I have lost over 30 pounds, my body fat has decreased, my lean body mass increased, and I have lost an amazing 20 inches from my abs, hips, thighs, and arms. I am closing in on my goal weight at this time. I have NEVER felt stronger and more alive. Rob, thanks for your expertise, skill, and encouragement. You have helped me put my life back together, and I will be forever and eternally grateful to you.

Are you still afraid to get started? Do you need a little more motivation? Do you think changing your body is unattainable? Have you gone through some tough times and need a pick me up? Read what Chris, who joined my women's only boot camp class a few years back, did.

In June of this year I received a postcard in the mail about a fitness boot camp for women. I thought it sounded like a great way to get in shape for a family wedding I had coming up. Little did I know what a great thing it would be for me! Not only was I feeling muscles I didn't know I had, but I was feeling great and had a ton of energy!

Looking back on the last 4 months, I realize that boot camp has also helped me in other ways of my life. I had a life-changing event happen to me and my three teenage sons in January of 2008. My husband of 22 years died suddenly of a heart attack at the age of 45.

After the shock wore off, I found myself not quite sure who I was. I wasn't a wife and a couple any more. I was a person who was the sole supporter of my family and realized that every decision I made was extremely important.

When Mike died, I told myself that I needed to take care of myself because my boys needed me to be there for them. I started making doctor appointments that I had put off and thinking about getting in shape. It seemed like an impossible task to find time to do everything.

When boot camp came along, there were no more excuses. What could I possibly be doing at 5:30 in the morning?! Rob and all the ladies at camp welcomed me and treated me as family. We work hard and have a lot of fun, too! I have found that the negative things I was thinking in my head have turned into positive things. Not only do I feel great, but I feel like I can try anything.

Rob has been an awesome influence in my life and an answered prayer.

Chapter 7: **Where do I start?**

Starting a fitness routine can be one of the most intimidating events in your life. You know that you want to get fit, but you just don't know what to do, and walking into a gym can scare the heck out of some people. I have talked to many women who said they drove in the parking lot on many different occasions before they actually walked through the front door of the fitness center.

There is a big misconception out there that other people are staring at you when you're new to a fitness facility. Believe me, this is a fallacy. The only reason people might be looking at you is because they never saw you before. Other than that, fitness is like a family, and everyone is excited for each other when they make a change to their physique or accomplish a fitness-related goal.

Everyone has to start somewhere, and, believe it or not, a good percentage of people who walk into a fitness facility have no clue as to what they are doing. Fitness has evolved, and we have found ways to get you results to change your body in a much quicker, easier fashion. You can even do it at home with minimal equipment.

I used to consult with women who played high school and college sports, and they would tell me, "Yeah, I know what to do, I played college volleyball." The more questions I asked, the more I realized that these women had no clue about what to do. Don't get me wrong; there are some women who have a good grasp on what to do, but this is definitely not the norm.

Typically, these women had practiced 2 to 3 hours per day and burned calories that way. Once they graduated and were taken out of their "normal training environment," they were as lost as the next person.

A woman named Katrina walked into my office the other day and said the same thing to me. If you were to see her in person, you would not think she needed any help getting in shape. However, she said "Rob, I played college soccer, but I'm intimidated to work out here." So we connected her with a professional trainer, and she is now looking fantastic. She is getting married this fall and should be proud of what she has accomplished in the gym. The biggest group of women that I have consulted with over the years is, believe it or not, is nurses. Yes, I am as shocked as you are.

Motivation is what gets you started;
habit is what keeps you going.

A few years ago, a lady named Kathryn joined our group. At boot camp, we always do fitness tests on the first and last Fridays so we can track results. It is always amazing how much improvement a person can make in a month. One of the tests is the mile run/walk. Kathryn hadn't run a mile in God-knows-how-long. She didn't think she could do it. She was approaching the final turn on the track, and several ladies who had finished already got up, ran over to her, and grabbed her to help finish the final 40 yards.

Tears nearly came to my eyes when I saw how powerful it is to work as a team and motivate each other. You will be happy to know that, since then, Kathryn has nearly cut her mile time in half—along with her body weight. She said something very profound: "People really treat you different when you're not fat." It's too bad that happens but pretty amazing that she transformed her body and now seems to have a much better outlook on things. Everyone has been asking about her, and she returns each summer.

The good news is that, once you absorb the information in this book, you will be able to start your own program at home, in the local park, or really anywhere you want. If you have questions, I will be here for you. You can contact me via email with any questions you may have from the information provided.

Chapter 8:   **Plan to succeed or you will fail**

I've seen it happen far more than I would like to admit. Many women start out with the greatest of intentions and then, like many other areas of life, just end up going through the motions. Life eventually gets in the way. They feel something is better than nothing. Many others feel that since they worked out today, it gives them a free ticket to go stuff down at their favorite garbage food joint.

I was working with one lady who, before I met her, weighed more than 300 pounds, taking diabetes medication, working out 7 days per week walking on a treadmill at a 15% grade for over an hour, burning 1,200 calories, and wondering why her body wasn't changing. After a little investigation, this gal was gobbling up over 1,800 calories after her work-out at the local fast food restaurant.

She had no plan and figured since she worked out so long and so hard, that it really didn't matter what she ate. Well, here is the good news! We got her on a plan to succeed.

She was already putting in the hard work, so I actually made her life easier by putting her on a simple plan of weight training and eating. She actually ended up working out less and got more time back for herself. She now understands that eating as much as she cared to eat after her workout wasn't the answer to her nutritional needs to help her transform her body.

Within a year and a half, she lost half of her body weight and no longer takes medication to control her diabetes. It doesn't have to be rocket science; you just need a simple plan that fits into your lifestyle, and then stick to it. Here are a few things you can start doing today to walk down the path to success.

1. Go grocery shopping once per week.

By doing this, you can be assured that you will be ready for the week. If you wake up and go into your cabinets and see nothing, it's not going to be a good day. The odds are that you will be visiting the enemy and eating something bad for you because you weren't prepared. Most of us know that we should not go grocery shopping on an empty stomach lest sugary treats start jumping into the shopping cart without our knowledge.

2. Plan your weekly meals.

It is important to know what you will be consuming for the next week. After a while, you will find yourself eating the same breakfasts, snacks and lunches and will only have to decide what dinner you will be having.

3. Pick one or two big cooking days.

Choose a day, usually Sunday works best, to cook up a large amount of your protein and complex carbs. This works well. You can then store the food in individual containers in the refrigerator. Presto, the hardest part of transforming your body is now done for a few days.

4. Create a workout log.

See the appendix for an example.

5. Journal your food.

Without question, this is the most useful tip for your success. This is what makes and breaks women's success. Whenever I have dealt with a woman that was starting to hit a wall on her body transformation, the first question I would ask is, "Are you still journaling your food?" Believe it or not, 100% of the time that I asked the question in this situation, the look on their face was like that of a puppy who knew it had done something wrong. The answer was always "no." Nowadays, there are so many free apps for your phone that can do this for you. They will even allow you to scan the barcode of the food, and it will enter all the data for you.

6. Set attainable goals, and write them down.

Trying to change your body without a goal is like going through a foreign city without a GPS. So many women who I have consulted with in the past have said, "I just want to get in shape" or "I want to get healthy." What does that mean? Either you don't know how to make a realistic goal or you are already setting yourself up just in case you fail. There is an acronym for setting goals called S.M.A.R.T. It stands for Specific, Measureable, Attainable, Realistic, and Timely. So make sure your goal meets these criteria. Once you have your goal, write it down, and put it somewhere you will see it every day. Set small goals regularly and reward yourself when your reach them.

7. Make sure you have a good support system.

Having people close to you that support your efforts is extremely important. One of my clients had told me that she works out 6 days per week and is having trouble changing her body. I told her that her eating habits are the issue, not the working out. She went on to say it's tough because her friends call her a "fuddy duddy" if she doesn't go out and drink with them. Is that a support system you want when trying to change your body? Surround yourself with people who have similar goals and interests when trying to transform.

8. Treat yourself once in a while. You are only human.

If you are eating well all week, a "cheat" meal once in a while will not ruin your success. The key is "once in a while." I had a lady tell me that she liked to entertain, so she drank alcohol only on the weekends. Her weekend started on Thursday. Think about it, she drank Thursday, Friday, and Saturday. It doesn't sound horrible until you realize that three days per week equates to 42% of the week during which she was getting toasted. That's almost half of her life!

Chapter 9:   The plan

The plan is really quite simple. There are three components needed for long-term body transformation. If ANYONE tells you they have a plan for you that doesn't incorporate ALL three, you will be set up for failure—guaranteed.

1. Boost your metabolism with resistance training.

2. Do cardiovascular training.

3. Eat clean, and don't starve yourself.

Chapter 10:

I don't want to bulk up, should I skip the weights?

As we will later touch on about metabolism, you will learn that weight training is a must for everyone, no matter your age or gender.

To all you women who are afraid of bulking up, it's not going to happen! Women don't have anywhere close to the amount of testosterone that men do. This is probably a good thing for many reasons. With that said, most men who are drug free aren't bulky, so don't fear the weight training. It is your ticket to a great body and a speedy metabolism.

A few years back while working out at the gym, I overhead two women talking about their lack of success with weights. Their story was quite interesting. (I always workout incognito; otherwise, I am shelled with questions. It's not that I mind answering questions, but on one occasion a lady tapped on my shoulder when I had a large amount of weight about to crush my chest, and she kept tapping until I looked up. I finished my rep and saved myself from almost having a heart attack from her startling me and almost crushing my chest with the weight on the bar.)

So, back to the story.

Two ladies were doing some very light dumbbell exercises right next to each other. I think I had counted about 29 repetitions before I lost track of how many reps they were doing. Then, one lady says, "This weight lifting stuff is useless, let's go do some cardio." The other lady agreed and, after probably 50 or more reps with their 3-pound weights, they put them back on the rack and left. I never saw them after that. I feel bad now as I probably should have chimed in and helped them out.

In order to get results with weight training, you have to push your body harder than it is used to being pushed. When you can do a movement more than 50 times, you may get tired, but you are not going to build any muscle to increase your metabolism. For example: You could swing a tennis racquet 50 times in a row and you probably would be tired; however, this isn't going to build quality muscle.

To keep it simple for beginners, you need to find a weight that allows you to do between 8 and 12 repetitions for 1 to 3 sets in a slow, controlled manner, with a 30-60 second rest in between. This is the range that will build the most muscle and lead you to that "toned" look. (But don't forget: Your eating habits will account for about 70% of how you look.)

One of the biggest mistakes I see women making is using this 8 to 12 repetition guideline as the holy grail. They stop the second they get to twelve reps, even if they could have done 13, 14, or more.

So, what would a "perfect" three sets look like? Set one, you have 10 pounds, do 14 reps, and can't do another one. Set two, you get to 11 reps before your arms feel like they are going to fall off. And set three, you get to 8 before you start screaming obscenities.

The next question might be, "How do I know when to increase my weights?" When those 10 pounds can be done well over the 12 reps for at least two of your three sets, it's time to jump to the next weight.

Chapter 11:
Can I really speed up my metabolism at any age?

When you look up the word "metabolism" in the dictionary, it reads, "the chemical changes in living cells by which energy is provided for vital processes and activities and new material is assimilated." Wow, it's really not that complicated, believe me. In laymen's terms, it translates to: how fast does the body process or burn through food.

Most women find that they can eat anything they want and not gain weight in their 20s and 30s, but, for some reason, once they hit that magic number of 40, things start to change. They tell me, "My metabolism slowed down once I hit 40." Does this sound familiar to you? I used to shake my head and chuckle when I heard this comment, and I heard it quite often. No, I wasn't being rude; it's just that comment has some partial truth but is very much avoidable.

There are research studies that show no correlation to age and declining metabolism in women as long as you are either doing intense cardiovascular training or resistance training. This research includes post-menopausal women and pre-menopausal women. Sedentary post-menopausal women had a lower metabolic rate than sedentary pre-menopausal women; however, age-related decline in resting metabolic rate was not observed in women who exercised regularly in either category. When understanding metabolism, you first need to realize that how much muscle tissue you have on your body is really what dictates your metabolism.

The more muscle you have, the faster your metabolism will be.

Think of your muscles as your body's furnace, and your body's fat as the coal. You put the coal (fat) into the furnace (muscle) to get burned up. So the more muscle that you have on your body, the more fat that you will be able to incinerate. Make sense?

When you eat food, the muscle will call for the food almost like a machine needing fuel. The more muscle you have, the more fuel needed, and the more fat that will get burned up in the muscle. For each additional pound of muscle you put on your body, you can expect to burn an extra 25 to 50 calories per day. This may not sound like much, but, considering that your body works seven days per week, if you added five pounds of lean muscle, you could potentially lose half of a pound per week for simply having extra muscle on your body. And let's not forget, you will look better, too.

Chapter 12:   Boost your metabolism

In order to burn fat, a few things need to happen: 1) fat needs to be released from the body, and 2) fat has to be transported to the muscle to be incinerated.

At this point, there is no magic pill that does both of these steps. Believe me, if there was a pill out there, I would probably tell you about it. I say "probably" because the odds are that the so-called magic pill would have so many side effects, I would probably need a separate book to list them. There are four sure-fire ways to boost your metabolism, however.

1. Eat often.

Eating three square meals a day is old hat when it comes to changing your body. The problem is that, when you eat just a few times per day, those few times turn into gorging feasts. When you eat often, you tend to eat less at each meal and are more energized throughout the day because you don't have crazy blood-sugar drops that make you hungry and sleepy. When it comes to your metabolism and eating, think of this campfire analogy. When you put 3 big logs on the fire (3 meals eaten per day), you smother the fire (you slow your metabolism down). When you put little pieces of kindling on the fire throughout the night (eat small meals throughout the day), you keep the fire burning hot (you stoke your metabolism).

2. Have protein at each meal.

Protein makes you feel full so you don't eat as much, and it helps repair muscles, which, in turn, can increase your metabolism (if you add lean muscle mass to your body from consistent resistance training). It can also do another little trick. It will cause your body to burn as much as 20% of the protein calories during digestion. Picture yourself putting a piece of chicken in your mouth and just letting it sit there. Not a lot happens. Now picture putting a cracker in your mouth. You will notice that the cracker starts to melt or digest. The body has no problem digesting the cracker and won't burn too many calories but has a difficult time breaking down the protein. The protein takes much more work to have it broken down. What a great trick that protein does! It's like a magician.

3. **Engage in HIIT.**

"HIIT" stands for High Intensity Interval Training. This type of training involves alternating between very intense bouts of exercise and low-intensity exercise. An example could be pushing yourself very hard on the elliptical for 30 seconds and then going at a slower pace for 60 seconds. This method can also be used with weights or any type of resistance equipment. The bonus to this activity that speeds up your metabolism is called the afterburn effect, or EPOC (Exercise Post Oxygen Consumption). You can burn calories for up to 24 hours after your bout of exercise. When you go for a typical jog, you burn close to zero calories after your workout.

4. **Add lean muscle mass.**

As noted above.

Chapter 13:   Don't sabotage your metabolism

There is one thing that can stop this whole fat-burning process from happening. No, it's not the gym being closed or your personal trainer being out of town. It's a bad man named sugar!

Many of us still pay attention to labels and jump up and down when we see 99% fat free. I think this has been ingrained in people's heads. However, the real bad boy is sugar. Excess sugar consumption can actually turn off your body's fat-burning abilities. If you are really interested in the details, you can research insulin and glucagon. To make a long story short, when you consume excess sugar, insulin is released, which aids in fat storage. When you keep sugar at bay and insulin is suppressed, a hormone called glucagon increases the breakdown of fats so you can be a fat burning machine.

Did you know that about 100 years ago, the average American consumed about 20 pounds of sugar per year, and a recent statistic showed that we are now close to consuming 150 pounds of sugar per year? I know statistics can lie to you, but the bottom line is that sugar consumption has gotten crazier than the cuckoo cocoa puffs bird.

Other things that can derail your success are:

• **Going on a "starvation diet"**

The 48-hour Hollywood diet, the grapefruit diet, the soup diet, et cetera. These types of diets starve your body. When this happens, you lose lean muscle mass, which means your metabolism drops and the weight will eventually come back at a much faster pace when you go back to your normal eating habits. See "the vicious cycle." You may know this better as yo-yo dieting.

• **Not working out.**

Did you ever hear the phrase, "If you don't use it, you will lose it"? Typically this is the case as women age. It's not that they eat more; it's that they aren't as active as they once were. If you don't use your muscles, they atrophy, or get smaller, and waste away. Muscle equates to metabolism, so you may stay the same weight but you lose muscle and gain fat.

• **Thyroid problem.**

Only about 3% of the population has a thyroid problem.

However, this can definitely put a stop to your fitness success if not treated properly. Your doctor can do some simple blood work to make sure that your thyroid is functioning properly.

Chapter 14:   How can I measure my metabolism?

Once you find out how many calories your body burns during the day, it makes it much easier to create a meal plan to reach your goals. You can then enter your meals into free online apps such as My Fitness Pal or Daily Burn to keep you on track.

There are several pieces of equipment at some gyms that can give you your daily resting metabolic rate with a high level of accuracy. We use the Korr metabolic tester at be fitness and wellness center in Delafield, Wis. I have seen other gyms use bodygem TM, which is pretty accurate as well.

Keep in mind that although getting your metabolism tested in nice, it is not necessary for transforming your body. By simply following a clean eating plan, doing strength training along with aerobic training, you will do just as well. It may just take a little more trial and error to fine tune your calorie plan. You can do this with the help of a few well-known formulas.

1. The simple rule of thumb

If you are looking to lose fat, plan on eating between 10 and 12 calories per pound of body weight. So, if you weigh 170 pounds, you would aim for about 1,700 calories. This is an average and can be over or underestimated based on you age and weight.

2. The Harris-Benedict formula

This formula is more scientific. It uses your height, weight, age and gender to determine your basal metabolic rate. This formula can be off if you have a very low activity level and a very high body-fat percentage. So, if you are very muscular of very obese, it may over or under estimate your calories.

3. The Katch-McArdle Equation

The Harris-Benedict equation has separate formulas for men and women because men usually have larger bodies and more lean body mass than women. Since the Katch-McArdle formula accounts for LBM, this single formula applies equally to both men and women. It's the most accurate method for calculating your daily caloric needs.

Chapter 15:
Cardiovascular activity... savior or enemy?

When most women join the gym or start a workout plan what is the first thing that goes through their minds? No, thinking about the cute trainer is not the answer I was looking for. Cardiovascular activity—hopping on the treadmill or elliptical or bike is typically a woman's first concern. Cardiovascular activity is definitely going to help you in the beginning to start burning off stubborn body fat, but it's not your number-one concern. If you don't have the muscle on your body to incinerate the fat, it could be a big waste of time.

When one of our highlighted women, Cheryl, was leaning out for her competition, she completely eliminated cardiovascular workouts and actually increased her calories because she was losing muscle and dropping far too much weight. From the previous chapter, you know how detrimental losing muscle mass can be to your metabolism, which affects your body transformation. Yes, I know this is a problem you would like to have, isn't it? Well, you can when you make your first priority strength training.

Remember Ann from earlier? She was one of my first clients who got off the elliptical machine bandwagon so she could start changing her body. She trusted me, and the word starting to spread at the gym. Women were finally starting to take the resistance-training portion of their workouts seriously.

We all know that both strength training and cardiovascular training are important. We also know that adding muscle mass improves your metabolism. I would like you to think about the following situation that exaggerates these concepts. Do you ever see a marathon runner who looks like a bodybuilder? No, this is because when you do so much cardiovascular training, your body starts to use muscle tissue for fuel.

Many marathon runners carry more body fat than normal athletes. They lose so much muscle mass, and, even though they run hundreds of miles, their metabolism is slowed down due to lack of muscle mass. I have personally seen many women long-distance runners look like they never even worked out and held body fat percentages above 30%, which is high for a sedentary individual. This is not true for everyone out there, but I see it more often than not for amateur runners.

So, be careful not to do too much cardio when trying to transform your body. How do you know how much is too much? You can have a fitness professional measure your body fat on a regular basis. This process will be able to tell you if you are losing muscle or body fat. If you are losing muscle, you are either not eating enough or doing too much cardiovascular training or a combination of both.

Many people ask, "Should I do my cardio or strength training first?" This all depends on your goal. For the sake of transforming your body, I suggest a 5- to 7-minute warm up, followed by strength training, followed by cardiovascular activity. (If you are training for a running event, I would suggest you do the cardiovascular training first.)

The theory is to get your strength in first because building your metabolism is of utmost importance. You'll get the most out of your strength workout by doing it first. If you choose to do your entire cardio workout first, you may not have the energy necessary to complete your strength routine, and your muscle gains won't be maximized.

Chapter 16:   How hard should I be working?

This is a question most women get wrong. It's not always about working harder, it's about working smarter. When it comes to your cardiovascular activity, if you push yourself too hard, you won't reap the benefits that you were initially out to get.

When you exercise, you should try to reach your training heart rate zone, and maintain it, for the duration of their aerobic activity. There are several methods to compute what your training heart rate should be.

Perceived exertion:

This method uses an intensity scale of 1 to 10, with 1 being very easy and 10 suggesting you are at 100% effort. Your goal is to aim for a 6, 7, or 8 on this scale. This scale is great for those who do not have a heart-rate monitor or those who take medications that control their heart rate.

220-age:

This is another simple method and somewhat outdated but still gives a fairly accurate starting point. Subtract your age from 220 and multiply by .65 (low end) and .85 (high end) and find a comfortable spot in between the two.

Example for a 30 year old

220-30=190

190 x .65 = 123 (this would be if you were out of shape)

190 x .85 = 161 (this is high intensity)

So your heart zone is between 123 and 161.

Karvonen formula:

This formula is considered to be a bit more accurate than just taking 220 minus your age. You can calculate your own training heart rate using the Karvonen Formula, but first you'll have to determine your Resting Heart Rate, Maximum Heart Rate and Heart Rate Reserve.

1. **Resting Heart Rate** (RHR) = your pulse at rest (the best time to get a true resting heart rate is first thing in the morning before you get out of bed).

2. **Maximum Heart Rate** (MHR) = 220-your age

3. **Heart Rate Reserve** (HRR) = Maximum Heart Rate - Resting Heart Rate

Once you have your Heart Rate Reserve, you can calculate your training heart rate:

4. **(Heart Rate Reserve *.85)** + Resting Heart Rate = Upper end of the training zone

5. **(Heart Rate Reserve *.50)** + Resting Heart Rate = Lower end of the training zone

Example: To calculate the training heart rate of a 35-year-old person with a resting heart rate of 70:

Maximum Heart Rate: 220-35=185 bpm (beats per minute)
Heart Rate Reserve: 185-70=115 bpm
High End of the Training Heart Rate: (115*.85)+70 = 167 bpm
Low End of the Training Heart Rate: (115*.50) +70 = 127 bpm

Many people have come to me and said, "On my treadmill at the gym, it says the fat-burning zone is closer to the low end of the training zone, so shouldn't I work out there for the best results?"

The so called fat-burning zone that you see on many pieces of equipment is often misleading. The theory is that if you work out at a lower intensity for a longer duration, you will burn more fat.

The reality is that while you may burn more fat calories, you will burn fewer calories overall, which means it will take you longer to reach you goal. So, when you feel like you are in good enough shape to workout at the higher end of your training zone, do it. The more calories burned equals the more fat lost.

Chapter 17:   Diets are for suckers, give them a kiss

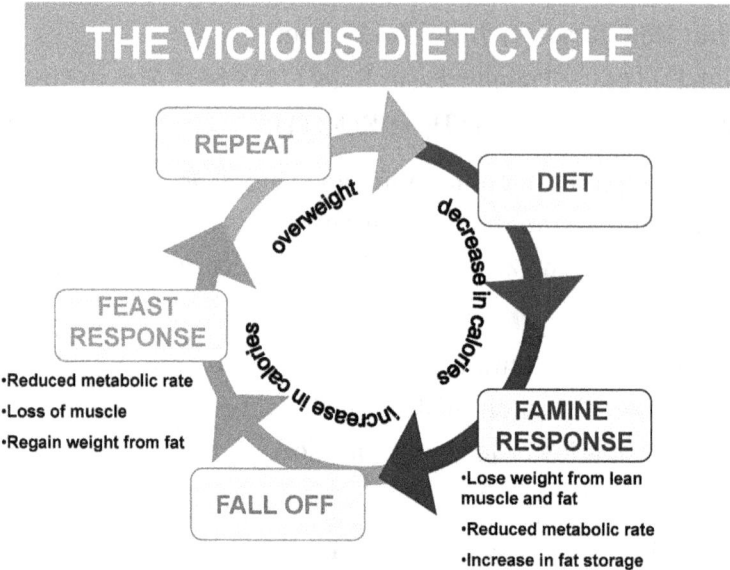

THE VICIOUS DIET CYCLE

REPEAT

DIET

overweight

decrease in calories

FEAST
RESPONSE

•Reduced metabolic rate
•Loss of muscle
•Regain weight from fat

increase in calories

FAMINE
RESPONSE

•Lose weight from lean
muscle and fat

•Reduced metabolic rate

•Increase in fat storage

FALL OFF

Have you been a victim of the vicious diet cycle?

I don't care what the latest and greatest research says out there; the second you see the word "diet," run for your life. A diet is never a lifestyle. It is always a restriction of what you can't do.

What's the first thing you want to do when someone tells you that you can't? When I was younger, my mother would tell me that I couldn't go to my grandparents' house without first shaving my face. Well, like most rebellious kids, that is what I was not going to do. I believe the same applies to food. If someone tells us we can't eat wheat or carbohydrates or my favorite dessert, cheesecake, it is the first thing we are going to want.

What comes to mind when you think of eating? Satisfaction? Feeling good? Fueling your body? What's for dessert?

What do you think of when you hear the word "diet"? Most people think quick, successful weight loss, feeling better, looking better. What you should really be thinking is that a quick fix will set you up for short-term success and eventual failure.

Almost every single diet out there will make you fall into the vicious cycle. A calorie-deprived "diet," regardless of the method, results in a temporary weight loss and usually the yo-yo effect, which means you will not only gain back the weight you lost but you will also get a bonus few pounds on top of where you started.

What do diets really do to you? Well, they certainly confuse you, for one. I think from here on out I should replace the word "diet" with the word "sabotage" because that's what they are. The problem is that a diet excites you because, when you look at the scale after a week or two, the number on the scale usually goes down. When the scale weight goes down that means you are successful, right? WRONG! This is the hardest thing for women to comprehend.

The weight you lose on a diet is typically water, muscle and very little fat. I had a client, Joanne, who, after about three months of working together had lost 10 pounds on the scale. She was disappointed in herself; however, she had dropped several dress sizes, lost 5% body fat, gained muscle, boosted her metabolism (so she could eat more food and still keep off the fat), and lost inches everywhere.

There was a demon in the room, and it was the scale.

All of the success she gained was overlooked by that dum-dum scale. If you take only one thing from this book, remember that the scale is a demon and can be misleading when it comes to changing your body. A pound of muscle is the size of a baseball, while a pound of fat is about the size of a brick. So, if you lose 5 pounds of fat and gain 5 pounds of muscle, your body will look so much better, yet the scale won't move one iota.

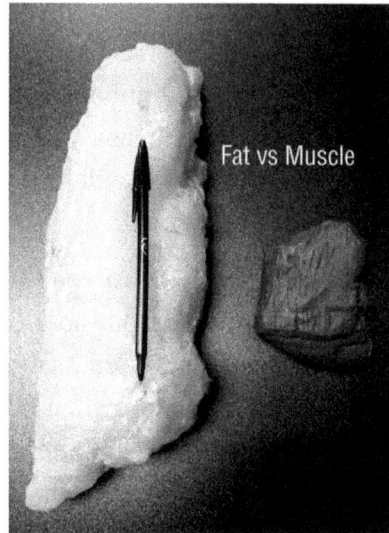

Fat vs Muscle

Concern yourself with how you look in the mirror or have a professional personal trainer take your body-fat percentage, as this is a much better indicator of your fitness success.

Let's discuss, in a bit more detail, the vicious diet cycle that nearly 100% of diets will take you through. First, you get excited because you heard about the new fad diet of the week. As I told you earlier, there certainly isn't a shortage of miracle diets out there. The next thing that happens is you follow your new diet to the letter.

What you don't realize is that there is no magic here; you are simply starving yourself to lose weight. You could be eating 1,000 calories of doughnuts, chips, soup or chocolate cake and still lose weight. You wouldn't feel good eating this junk, but you won't feel good starving yourself either. If losing weight and changing your body is so easy, then why are there so many books out there? And why are we obese as a nation?

Well, let's start with the first part. It's not hard to lose weight. It's keeping the weight off part that tends to be the hardest, because when you lose the weight, do you really know what you lost? I'm guessing mostly water, muscle and a little bit of fat, but your friend the scale doesn't know this information. The scale just shows that you have lost weight. So the next thing that happens is a feeling of success and excitement.

The real problem is what's happening behind the big curtain. What is the wizard really doing back there? You are starving yourself which leads to losing lean muscle mass. This plan is setting you up for failure and you don't even know it— and that's the icing on the chicken breast. It's not your fault, your program is failing you.

When you lose muscle mass, your metabolism drops, which means you now have to eat less food to lose weight. That certainly doesn't sound good, does it? As you keep starving, you continue to lose "weight" (mostly muscle mass) and your metabolism continues to drop. So you come to a point where the weight loss stops. What happens next? Well, they take more food away from you. So now all you can eat in a day is a forkful of chicken and two peas due to your drastic drop in metabolism.

The thought now racing through your head is that you just aren't cut out for this type of diet. You quit, go on a binge for a weekend, and fall into a food coma. The weekend binge continues until you wake up, gain all the weight back (and a few extra pounds), find the next diet on the shelf, and start the process all over again.

The funny-but-not-so-funny thing about this cycle is that if you ask any women about their diet plan, they will say it was a success and would encourage anyone to give it a shot. They will go on to tell you that they are going to do it again themselves.

How can something be a success if it failed you? I consider a success when you reach your goal and can maintain it, not gain twice as much weight back before you started the diet.

Chapter 18:   Will eating wheat affect my results?

There's no evidence that a gluten-free diet helps with weight loss. It really depends on the choices you make. If you replace foods that contain gluten with whole foods like fruits and vegetables, you may successfully lose weight. On the other hand, if you replace them with gluten-free packaged foods, you probably won't experience much success. Most of these foods are made with refined flour, and some even add sugar and other ingredients that defeat the purpose. Going gluten-free is no magic bullet when it comes to transforming your body. Don't get caught up in the hype. You may even end up gaining weight.

Eating wheat or wheat gluten will not stop anyone's transformation from being a success. As a matter of fact, all of the women that were successful ate some form of wheat in their meals at some point. This new craze of cutting out wheat and going gluten free is not much different than the 10 million other low-carb diets out there, the newest, or I guess I could say oldest, being the "paleo diet."

When you take out major food items that most people eat and replace them with lower-calorie foods, of course you initially lose weight because you are cutting out a major portion of your calories. Wheat has been shown to have some inflammation properties internally in the body, and most processed wheat does have a higher glycemic index if eaten by itself.

My advice is always to eat in moderation. Is cutting out wheat totally necessary? Maybe for those people who are allergic to gluten, but not for transforming your body. Did all of our body-transformation women eat some wheat products? Yes, they did.

There is a lot of talk out there about wheat causing heart disease and other problems because wheat is now genetically modified. I'm not going to get in the middle of this one. One of our inspirations, Cheryl, recently had her blood work done and had impressive HDL numbers and very low LDL and triglycerides with no worries of her blood-glucose levels.

I think we sometimes forget that when we are overweight, our triglycerides, which are stored in our adipose tissue, will be high. But, no wheat to lose weight? You might as well say no carbs to lose weight.

I have said it many times, diet equals restriction, and restriction equals short-term success. For some people, a diet that's free of gluten isn't a choice—it's a necessity. However, why do people who don't have celiac disease go gluten free? One reason is they believe it will help them lose weight.

From a health standpoint, some people don't have a choice when it comes to giving up gluten from their daily food intake. If you've been diagnosed with celiac disease, following a gluten-free diet is a "must" to control intestinal inflammation but not a must for the rest of us to lose weight and transform.

If you are set on transforming your body and eliminating wheat at the same time, some good carbohydrate alternatives to wheat you can try are sprouted or sourdough bread, brown rice, quinoa, millet oats, and "dry" beans. Other healthier carbs include sweet potato, winter squash and lower-GI fruits such as berries. These healthier choices came from registered dietician and friend of mine, Pamela Voelkers.

Chapter 19: A calorie isn't just a calorie

In my experience, you can find a study to back anything that you want. I'm sure there is a study out there that shows doughnuts are the next magic pill to lose weight! Out of all of this hype and controversy, there is one thing that I believe in, and that is that a calorie isn't just a calorie. It just makes a lot of common sense, and here's why.

Harvard researcher Rachel Carmody is calling for the Atwater system, which is used to determine caloric values, to be updated. She says the calorie values reported on food labels do not capture costs of digestion. Protein foods can burn 20% to 30% of the food's calories during digestion, while fats only burn about 3% of the food during digestion.

We call that the thermic effect of food. So although two foods might have the same number of calories on the label, these calories are not equally available to the body depending on the marco-nutrients (proteins, carbs, and fats).

In addition to the thermic effect of food, healthy, clean foods in their natural state have been shown to burn more calories, while processed foods prepared in different ways burn fewer calories when digested.

In another study by the Harvard Medical School, a low-glycemic-index diet (eating clean foods) showed an increase in metabolism without any negative side effects. The study suggests that the low-glycemic load is more effective than conventional approaches at burning calories at a higher rate after weight loss. And this is when the comparable diets have the same amount of calories.

Chapter 20:   **Eat, eat, and eat to lose fat**

If you can follow a clean eating plan 90% of the time, you will be amazed at what you can accomplish. What exactly does "eating clean" mean? It's really simple. If it comes in a box, a wrapper, or if the label is filled with more than a few ingredients, then back the truck up and stay away.

A clean eating plan includes a lean, protein, complex carb, and fibrous vegetable at every meal or snack. In a nutshell, eat whole, natural foods (such as vegetables), lean proteins (such as chicken or fish), and complex carbohydrates (such as brown rice or sweet potatoes).

When I say chicken or fish, I'm not talking about a fish fry or deep-fried chicken. You would be surprised! I was once discussing eating habits with a female client who wanted to lose fat, and she was telling me how well she ate. She had chicken and fish and vegetables all the time. I was having a hard time figuring out where she was going wrong until she let me know that the chicken and fish were fried fast food. She honestly thought that since she was eating chicken, regardless of how it was prepared, that she was doing a good job.

An easy way to remember if a food is clean is: "If man made it, don't eat it." Additionally, when it comes to transforming your body, I would rather see you eat more vegetables than fruits.

Simple clean eating guidelines:

• Eliminate refined sugars and flour
• Limit dining out unless you are in the kitchen preparing the

meal because you just don't know what is being used for preparation

• Drink a lot of clean water (a good rule of thumb for beginners is half your body weight in ounces per day)

• Eat often during the day (every 3 to 4 hours)

• Consume a lean protein, starchy carb, and vegetable at each meal

• Eliminate alcoholic beverages

• Eat healthy fats such as omega 3's

• If it wasn't around 100 years ago, don't eat it

Eating clean can be a major transition for a majority of people due to addictions to sugar, white bread, and fast food. It takes discipline to make eating clean a habit, but it is possible and has many long-term health benefits. Try to follow the 90/10 rule. Eat good food 90% of the time, and allow yourself to indulge 10% of the time. This way of thinking will allow you to stay sane and never be deprived of what you like.

You can have your cake and eat it, too; just don't eat the entire cake, and don't get into a habit of doing it every day. Set a day to look forward to having your favorite food.

Eating clean table of "1st tier" of foods

Proteins:	Chicken Breasts
Lean or Extra Lean Ground Turkey	Organic Eggs
Egg Whites	Grass-Fed Beef
Wild-Caught Salmon	Tuna
Most white fish	Whey protein powder/protein bars

2nd tier- Milk, dairy, cheese, yogurt, cottage cheese

Carbs/Starches:	Oatmeal
Brown Rice	Quinoa
Sweet Potatoes	Legumes
Steel cut oats	Oat flour
Rolled oats	Peas

2nd tier- whole grain pastas, breads, tortillas, bagels, English muffins, Pitas, pancakes, rice

*Carbohydrates are not your enemy. An overabundance of calories is!

Vegetables:	Broccoli
Cauliflower	Kale
Spinach	Red peppers
Asparagus	Green beans
Zucchini	Eggplant
Brussels sprouts	Onions

Healthy Fats:	Natural Peanut Butter
Almond Butter	Walnuts
Pistachios	Sunflower seeds
Avocado	Olive Oil
Grape seed Oil	

Miscellaneous:

Sweeteners: Stevia

*This list is in no way all-inclusive but just a starting point.
*Remember just because some fats are good for you, it doesn't meant that you can consume as much as you want of them. Too much of anything will make you fat!

An example of 1,500-calorie clean eating plan

50% carbohydrates, 30% protein, and 20% fat

Breakfast

Egg white omelet (4 egg whites, ½ cup diced tomatos, a touch of water)

1 cup oatmeal

Lunch

*This is an example and not a prescription.

1C Brown Rice

3oz Chicken breast

1/3 C black beans

1 C mixed vegetables

Snack

1 C Almond milk

½ C Blueberries

1 Scoop Protein powder (approximately 20g)

Dinner

3oz Salmon

2 C asparagus

1TBL olive oil

Eating the right amount of calories is important, but even more important is the percent of macronutrients and the ability to eat throughout the day. To be successful, you can't use the old adage of eating three square meals per day or think that because that you only ate once per day that you will lose unwanted body fat.

Typically, I prefer one of three different eating plans when it comes to transforming a woman's body. But before I go into the plans, it is important to figure out how many calories your body needs to reach your goals.

Use one of the methods explained earlier to get your daily calorie needs for transformation. (The formulas are in the appendix) When that is completed, we will subtract 10% to 15% of the caloric intake to start losing that stubborn fat. The key is not to go into such a deficit where you start to lose too much muscle. So, never drop below a 30% deficit, and never drop below 1,200 calories without a medical professional's supervision.

1. *I'm ready phase 1.*

This phase is set up to get women used to eating more meals spaced throughout the day with a good combination of carbohydrates, proteins, and fats. It is set up with a proper calorie count to get women reading labels and measuring what they eat. With the correct calorie count, every woman will start to lose weight. The General Daily Macronutrient percentages are 50% Carbohydrates, 30% Protein, and 20 % fat.

2. *Get me hot phase 2.*

This phase will get most people to reach their transformation goals. You can start at this phase if you want to reach your goals quicker and have the motivation to keep you going. It adds more protein for satiety and muscle building. The small drop of carbohydrates is usually enough for most people to start seeing some serious fat loss and extra protein will help building and maintaining muscle mass for metabolism. The breakdown of macronutrients is this phase is: 40% protein, 40% carbohydrates, 20% fat.

Note: When you read about Cheryl, note that she got in fitness-competition shape using phase 2 for her entire program. She went on the Phase III plan for one week and started to drop too much body fat. She was entering a fitness competition where you don't want a lot of veins sticking out. Phase 2 put her at 8% body fat in less than 12 weeks. You can read about her meal plans, supplements and workouts later on.

3. *Rip it off me phase 3* (carb cycling).

This phase tricks the body into losing fat yet holding onto your gains. It is used to lose the last few stubborn body fat percentages, if needed. It consists of 3 days of protein and mostly vegetables at a 15-20% calorie deficit, followed by one day of protein and some starchy carbohydrates at a 15-20% surplus above your daily energy needs. Note this phase is advanced. Most women will have no problem getting to where they want to be with phase one or two.Macro nutrients for days 1-3 on this program are as follows: 25% carbohydrates, 45% protein, and 25% fat. Day four's macronutrients would be 50% Carbohydrates, 30% Protein, and 20 % fat.

Note: Mary used phase 3 during the last month of her training, and the last two weeks she just did the first part of phase 3, which means she did protein and vegetables with minimal starchy carbohydrates earlier in the day. You can see her entire plan later on.

Chapter 21: **Nutrition 101 "Marcos"**

With all the talk about macronutrients and calories, I think it's important to give you a little information about what they are and what they do before you make your own eating plan. Talking about macronutrients, vitamins, and minerals could very easily be a book by itself. One of my goals in this book is to keep things simple, so let's see how I do.

There are three major macronutrients (and an additional one that is only important if you frequent the local watering hole too much, and, if you're doing that, you probably aren't ready to make a change).

1. Protein
2. Carbohydrates
3. Fat
4. Alcohol

Protein is found in meat, poultry, fish, legumes, eggs, protein powders, nuts, seeds, milk, grains, and small amounts in some fruits and vegetables. Vegetarians will need more assistance to make sure they are eating complete proteins. Getting enough protein will help build and preserve muscle tissue when combined with a resistance training program. Protein makes you feel full, fights off appetite, and burns the most calories during digestion.

1 gram of protein=4 calories

Carbohydrates are the body's preferred energy source. They are stored in the liver and muscles. An overabundance of carbohydrates in the body is stored as fat. Carbohydrates are found in rice, potatoes, milk, bread, fruits, vegetables, legumes and many processed foods such as chips and soda. If you starve yourself and run out of carbohydrates, the body will break down your muscles to make fuel. This is what most diets do; hence you lose muscle mass and lower your metabolism. Don't fear the carbs!

1 gram of carbohydrates = 4 calories

Fat is essential to human life. It provides energy, absorbs nutrients, and helps insulate the body.

1 gram of fat = 9 calories, over 2 times that of proteins and carbohydrates

Alcohol dehydrates the body at the cellular level, removes inhibitions, increases your appetite, and decreases your reaction time. Alcohol is like rocket fuel, meaning that when you consume alcohol, all other nutrients are spared, and alcohol becomes the primary fuel. This means that the food you eat gets stored as fat while your body sucks up the suds.

1 gram of alcohol = 7 calories

So how do we figure this info out on a nutrition label?

Well, as discussed:

> 1 gram fat = 9 calories
>
> 1 gram protein = 4 calories
>
> 1 gram carbohydrate = 4 calories

Vitamins and minerals are micronutrients and do not contain calories. So, no, vitamins don't give you energy; food does.

A quick label reading

So whether you want to figure out how many calories or how many grams of each macronutrient you need, you now have the tools. Let's take a look at a nutrition label to see how it all works.

This product has 230 calories. Make note that this is for 2/3 cup serving, not the entire product. Sometimes when you look at a product, you may think it is for the entire container, but that is probably not the case. This is a tricky little thing to make some people think that they are eating less than they really are.

So 8 grams fat x 9 calories per gram= 72 calories from fat. 72 / 230 = 31% fat

37 g carbohydrate x 4 cal per gram= 148 calories from carbs. 148/230=65% carbs

3 g protein x 4 calories per gram= 12 calories from protein. 12/230=5% protein

Add up the calories, and you get the approximate total per serving,

The % daily value of fat, carbs, and protein, is based on a 2,000-calorie eating plan, so it doesn't have much value unless your plan recommends 2,000 calories. The percentages of vitamins

Nutrition Facts

Serving Size 2/3 cup (55g)
Servings Per Container About 8

Amount Per Serving

Calories 230	Calories from Fat 72

	% Daily Value*
Total Fat 8g	**12%**
Saturated Fat 1g	**5%**
Trans Fat 0g	
Cholesterol 0mg	**0%**
Sodium 160mg	**7%**
Total Carbohydrate 37g	**12%**
Dietary Fiber 4g	**16%**
Sugars 1g	
Protein 3g	

Vitamin A	10%
Vitamin C	8%
Calcium	20%
Iron	45%

* Percent Daily Values are based on a 2,000 calorie diet. Your daily value may be higher or lower depending on your calorie needs.

	Calories:	2,000	2,500
Total Fat	Less than	65g	80g
Sat Fat	Less than	20g	25g
Cholesterol	Less than	300mg	300mg
Sodium	Less than	2,400mg	2,400mg
Total Carbohydrate		300g	375g
Dietary Fiber		25g	30g

and minerals is based on the amount you need daily to avoid diseases, such as scurvy from lack of vitamin C.

Guide for making your daily food plan

1. Invest in a food scale to correctly measure and weigh your food.

2. Find your daily caloric needs using one of the methods mentioned earlier.

3. To lose fat/weight, deduct 10-20 % of the total daily caloric needs.

4. Decide which proportions you will use for the macronutrients (proteins, carbs, and fats). For example, phase 2 calls for 40% carbohydrates, 40% protein, 20% fat.

5. Choose how many meals per day you will be eating (4-6).

6. Divide total calories needed per day for weight loss by the number of meals per day to figure out how many calories you should consume at each meal. (For example, 1500 calories, 5 meals per day = 300 calories per meal.)

7. Figure out the total grams of protein/carbs/fat at each meal. (For example, 300 calories of protein per day/4 grams per calorie= 75 grams per day /5 meals = 15 grams of protein each meal. Remember fat has 9 calories per gram, protein and carbs have 4 calories/gram.)

8. Choose a lean protein, starchy carb, and fibrous vegetable for each meal.

EXAMPLE:

Daily calorie needs = 1500 calories

Weight loss deficit of 10% = 150 calories

New daily needs for weight/fat loss= 1350

Using phase 2 which is 40% protein, 40 % carbohydrate, and 20 % fat

Protein needs (40% protein = 1350 calories x .40 = 540 calories from protein)

Each gram of protein = 4 calories

540 calories /4 = 135 grams of protein for the day

135 grams/4 meals per day = 33 grams of protein per meal

Protein calories per day	Grams of protein per day	Grams of protein per meal
540	135	33

Carbohydrate needs (40% carbohydrates= 1350 calories x .40 = 540 calories from carbohydrates)

Each gram of carbohydrate =4 calories

540 calories /4 = 135 grams of carbohydrates per day

135 grams/ 4 meals per day = 33 grams of carbohydrates per meal

Carbohydrate calories /day	Grams of carbs per day	Grams of carbs per meal
540	135	33

Fat needs, 20% fat (1350 calories x .20= 270 calories from fat)

> Each gram of fat = 9 calories
>
> 270 calories/9= 30 grams of fat per day
>
> 30 grams /4 meals per day = 8 grams of fat per meal

Fat calories per day	Grams of fat per day	Grams of fat per meal
270	30	8

9. If choosing Phase 3, choose a lean protein and fibrous vegetable for days 1-3. On day 4, choose a lean protein, starchy carb and fibrous vegetable. Days 1-3 have a 10-20% deficit, and day four has a 10-20% surplus of calories.

Chapter 22: Fast food won't get you "phat" results

Americans spent $165 billion in fast food in 2010.

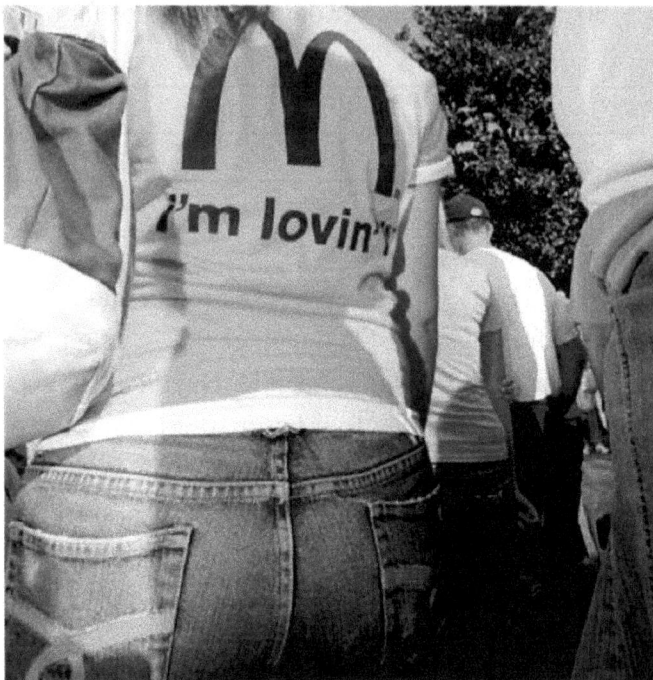

Do some of these places really need to be open 24 hours?

There is so much convenience out there these days that can wreak havoc on your eating plan. When I was growing up, it was a treat to get to go out for fast food maybe once or twice per month. Nowadays, it's the norm to go out a few times per week for either breakfast, lunch, or dinner. And let's not forget the 1,000-calorie coffees that are available to us at all hours. On top of that, let's take a look at the calorie kings out there. A hamburger used to be a little snack, but over the past 20 years, it has turned into a feast.

Cheeseburger

20 Years Ago

Today

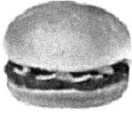

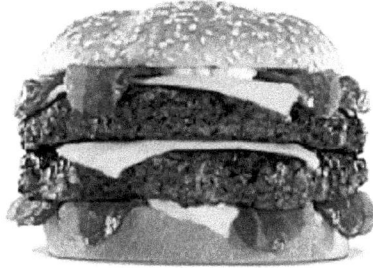

333 Calories

1,420 Calories

Calorie Difference: 1,087 calories

As consumers, we aren't happy if we don't get our money's worth when we go out to eat, which typically means the plate is stacked so high that you can't see the person across from you.

Portion control has gone wild. At one national Italian food chain, you are served six servings of pasta with your order. Let's not forget that these noodles are hanging out in a vat of oil before you get your lips on them. Most entrees have far more than you and your date would need for an evening out or an entire day for that matter. We all think chicken is healthy right? Try Olive Garden's Chicken Alfredo, it's only 1,440 calories and 82 grams of fat.

I recently read that McDonald's will discontinue offering apples with kids' meals. I guess the French fries have them hooked. Most of these places have an alternative healthy choice to pick, but they just aren't as appealing as their deep-fried counterparts. As a matter of fact, for a limited time in 2013 and at select locations in Japan, you could get a container of fries so big that it's officially the most caloric container of fries that any McDonald's has ever offered.

Called the "Mega Potato," the 350-gram serving of fries comes in a movie screen-wide cardboard container and weighs in at about 1,150 calories. This is close to what the typical women should be consuming as far as calories go for an entire day, and some people are eating this as part of a meal!

There are healthy choices when you dine out, but you really have to look for them. You usually can't go wrong at most sub places, and almost everyone offers a salad nowadays. Just make sure you know what's in the salad, because they can be very sneaky.

There was a study done on a college campus. For one semester, the girls ate at the salad bar every day while the guys the hamburgers, hot dogs, et cetera, in the hot food line. At the end of the semester, guess who gained the most weight. I'm sure it's pretty obvious right? The girls gained the most weight. They had a grand ole time adding croutons, cheese, high-calorie salad dressing, and anything else they could throw on top of those poor old lettuce leaves.

Did you know one of those little salad dressing containers hold 3 tablespoons, which, if it is a normal dressing, would equate to 45 grams of fat just from the salad dressing alone. You might as well have had the cheeseburger and fries.

Chapter 23:   How badly do you want it?

Did you hear the story about the young man who approaches a guru? The young man asks the guru what is the secret to being successful. The guru says, "If you want to know the secret, meet me at the beach tomorrow at 4 a.m." The young man thinks he is crazy but, nonetheless, shows up to the beach at 4 a.m. in his suit and tie. The guru is out in the water and waves the young man to walk out to him. The upset young man says, "I came here for a lesson on success not swimming."

The young man walks out to his waist, decides to turn around, and starts walking back towards the beach. The guru says, "I thought you wanted to be successful," and the young man says, "I do." The guru tells the young man to walk out to him again. At this point, the guru is shoulder deep in the water. As the young man gets closer, the guru grabs his head and pushes it down in the water. The young man gulps some seawater as he goes down.

The guru holds him down for about 20 seconds, and, just before the young man is about to go unconscious, the guru lets go. When the young man pops his head up, the guru says, "I have a question for you. When I had your head down in the water, what was the only thing that you were thinking about?" The young man said that he wanted to breathe. The guru said, "When you want to succeed as badly as you want to breathe, you will be successful!"

How badly do you want to be successful in your fitness transformation? Don't miss the opportunity to make a dream become reality.

Chapter 24:   **We don't plateau, we keep getting better.**

Almost all of the time when a client has hit a wall, I ask them if they are still journaling their food. Guess what? 100% of the time, the answer is 'no.' Once we get the eating plan back on track, the body responds.

The key to continually getting results is to keep things fresh. You need to change up some of the variables of your program. When it comes to the workouts, you can change the weight being lifted, the exercises being performed, the number of sets completed, the rest periods, etc.

Your body is very smart and adapts quickly to the things you do. Not only does your body adapt, but, if you continue to lift heavy weights without a break, your body will most likely break down and get injured.

I recommend changing some variables of your program every four to eight weeks. (See the periodization chart in appendix.) This applies to both your cardiovascular plan as well as your resistance-training program. When doing your cardiovascular plan, the body gets more efficient. A workout that may have burned 500 calories a few months ago may only burn 50 today. It is always important to mix it up, just like anything in life.

I have had many aerobics instructors come to me and ask what is wrong with them. They teach the same class three days per week and follow a balanced food program and their body isn't changing. The main problem is that they teach the same class. What started out as a calorie-burning monster eventually becomes the equivalent exercise of chewing a piece of gum. Well, not quite, but you get the idea.

Changing it up can also mean trying something different. Train for a 5K mud run, or try kickboxing or Zumba. You will never know until you try. Nothing ventured, nothing gained, right?

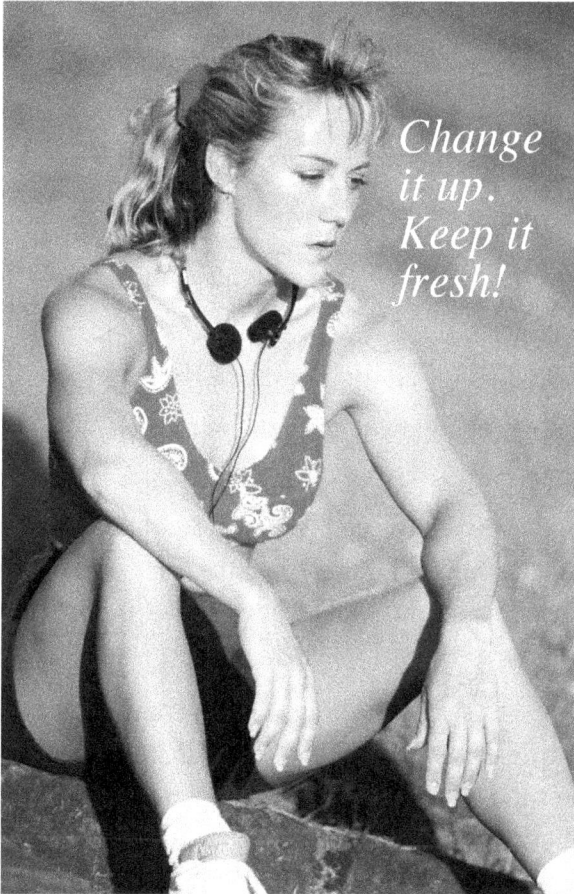

Change it up. Keep it fresh!

Chapter 25:   Words from a Master

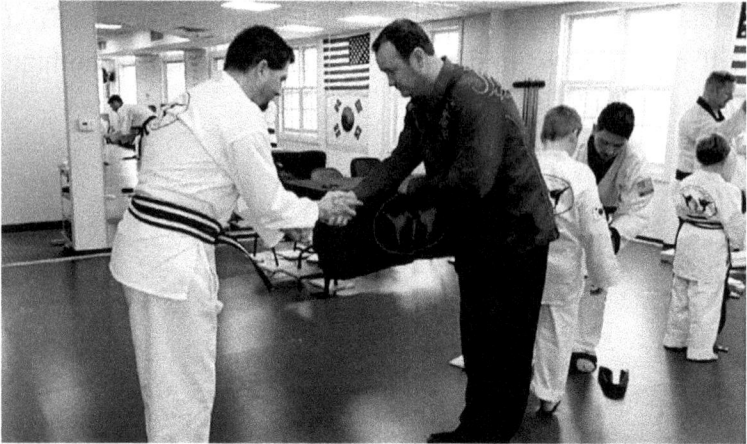

It's easy to be comfortable, but it doesn't get you results in the long term. Working out is only as challenging as you make it. I can give you the tools, but I can't make you try harder or make you come to boot camp.

If you always walk to a station, try jogging to it. If you have been using 5-pound weights, try 7 or 8 pounds. A little competition can be a good thing. Give the fastest runner in your class a challenge, and make them prove that they are the fastest. This type of attitude helps everyone.

People need to step out of their comfort zones. I realize we all have different levels of fitness, but that doesn't mean you can't use someone else to motivate you to do more than you are used to doing.

Tae Kwon Do Master Instructor Nick Elliott talks about life after every class. Recently, he talked about becoming complacent. He said, "Life is continuous, not ending. You have so many opportunities, so don't stop."

When he became a fifth-degree black belt, he was considered a master instructor. He could have stopped there. Instead, he earned his sixth-degree black belt last month. The 38-year-old has his future in martial arts all planned out: He will be a ninth-degree black belt when he is 62.

"You need to constantly think about how you can get better," he says. Even when he gets to ninth degree, that won't mean he's done. He will go back and see what he can improve. Just because he will have accomplished the highest degree doesn't mean that he is the best at tae kwon do. There are always people who are better.

"Ask yourself, 'How can I get better? What can I get better at?' Then write these things down and start to work toward them," he says. Having these types of goals is what drives people.

Master Elliott compares complacency to waddling with turkeys—you're with everyone else making noise. "You need to break away, make goals, and lay down the groundwork for leaving your legacy. There's a reason eagles soar alone. It's hard to be at their level. Waddling with turkeys is easy. You simply do what you have always been doing," he explains.

He emphasizes that success starts with you, not because someone else wants you to change. The key is to do one thing at a time. If you apply what you have learned, then you will start to see results, and, when you see results, you will start to gain confidence. You will talk better about yourself, and having a positive mindset is key.

Master Elliott sees himself as a leader. "If I'm not helping my students, then I shouldn't be up there (teaching) every day," he says. He's always thinking, "How can I motivate these people to do their best and be the best they can be? I need to practice what I preach. If I was overweight and told students to lose weight, they would think I was silly," he says.

He knows that everyone has personal struggles and obstacles in life. There is a time to cry, a time to laugh, and a time to get angry, but don't let these emotions take over your life. "Cry when you're sad, but don't get stuck in that place. We can all take negative experiences and find light," he says.

One of the biggest struggles in his life was an accident he had at age 17. His leg was burned to the point where doctors thought they would have to amputate at the knee. He was not going to let that happen. He stayed positive and took a chance with an experimental surgery.

He made it through but his girlfriend left him. It was a tough time, and he could have had a pity party, but he knew that wouldn't get him anywhere. During the next twenty years, he has accomplished many things because he decided not to waddle with the turkeys. He wanted to make a positive impact in people's lives.

"Anytime you try something new, you will face pitfalls. That's just the way it is," he says. Master Elliott says consistency is the best way to stay on track.

"Don't wake up at 5 o'clock and work hard one morning; get a schedule. Take yourself out of your comfort zone, and try to be consistent. You're not going to feel like working out every day. This is where discipline comes into play. Discipline is doing what you are supposed to do when you are supposed to do it. Make appointments for success just like you make appointments for the doctor," he says.

You need to give 100% every day. When approaching your workout, don't think about the problems of the day or what your kids need at school. Stay focused on the task at hand.

"Life boils down to what decisions you make on an hour-to-hour basis," he says. "The only way you can change is by making different decisions," he adds. You will be surprised at what your body can do once you convince your mind that it is possible. Your fitness destiny is in your hands.

Chapter 26:   Don't worry about falling off the wagon

Too many people get complacent and have a hard time staying with it. Even on the popular dramatic weight-loss TV shows, many people gain the weight back because what they did to get there simply doesn't fit into their lifestyle. They were not living in reality by having a personal chef and trainer on a daily basis. You can learn tricks of the trade from ordinary people of all ages who live a real life, not some dream portrayed on a TV show.

No matter what your age, you literally have no excuse. Your body didn't fall apart over night, and it's not going to become sculpted overnight. So be consistent, follow the guidelines, and don't make it more difficult than it really is. Research shows that if you can keep the weight off and maintain a healthy weight for five years, you have a 90% chance of keeping it off for good.

However, the reality is that you will face struggles. Life will get in the way, and things won't ever be perfect. You will stumble more than once. The key is to get up more times than you fall down.

Failure is how we continually learn and improve. Almost all successful people fail. Look at Michael Jordan; he got cut from his high school basketball team. That didn't stop him from becoming arguably the best basketball player of all time. When Thomas Edison was working on the light bulb he allegedly said, "I have not failed 1,000 times. I have successfully discovered 1,000 ways to NOT make a light bulb."

There is no roadmap for life, but the more we learn, the easier things will be for us in the future. I remember reading a popular book called "Tuesdays with Morrie." When Morrie was old and dying, he was asked if he could be 20 again, would he do it. His response was that if he were 20, he wouldn't have all the knowledge that he had at that day. He got wiser with every day on this earth.

Continue to gain knowledge, and keep it simple. Don't make this transformation tougher than it really is. As you read through some of these women's journeys, I'm sure you will see yourself in some of their situations. Learn from their mistakes, and take advantage of their tips for success.

Chapter 27:
I guess we don't learn everything in Kindergarten

I remember seeing an old poster that stated everything you need in life you learned in kindergarten. Well, I learned a few more things at Waterford High School's 2014 graduation ceremony. It sure is amazing how lessons learned in high school relate not only to life in general but to fitness and transformation in particular.

The salutatorian mentioned how people say you need to figure out how to love and be happy after graduation. You will notice that you will have a tough time completing a body transformation if you don't love yourself. You absolutely 100% need to do this for you. When you transform yourself for yourself, from within, you will feel not only a sense of accomplishment but also happiness.

Fitness is one of the only fields I know that when you are successful, no one can take it away from you. People might say, "Oh, he got that job because he knows the owner of the company" or "They drive that nice car because they inherited a lot of money." There is nothing anyone can say to take your success away when you change your body. You did it all by yourself.

You took the information and applied it. You choose the turkey breast when you could've had the meatball sandwich. You chose to work out when others chose to go out. You decided to make it happen while others watched it happen. You did it, and they wished they had. It feels pretty good when you make it happen. Be aware, when you are on top, you will still unfortunately encounter some naysayers.

Many people will be jealous and try to sabotage your efforts. You will see who your true friends are.

During the speech, the student also talked about measuring success not by salary, grade point average, or number of likes of a selfie (did you know that the word "selfie" actually made it into the dictionary in 2014?) but rather by the number of lives we touch. As I hope some of our stories touch your life, I also hope you will be able to pay it forward by motivating someone else to get fit, change their body, and change their life.

Now that you have your blueprint for success, remember that you have to do the work.

I was lucky enough to attend an NFL Hall of Fame induction ceremony for two former Green Bay Packers, Ahman Green and Ken Ruettgers. During their speeches, both gentlemen stressed the importance of hard work and dedication in obtaining their success. The average professional football career is about four years, and, with this in mind, they must put absolutely everything they have into those few short years.

So, now it's your turn. Take your plan, put in the effort, and you will be successful in your journey. A few points to consider as you begin:

Make sure you're ready

Do it for you

Don't make it more complicated than it really is.

Stay dedicated and work hard

Touch some lives and let people touch your life

Be a role model

Love yourself

If you fall down, get back up. Giving up is not an option

Never stop learning

When you face adversity, you have two choices, let the event define you or you define the event.

Your dream is out there; go get it.

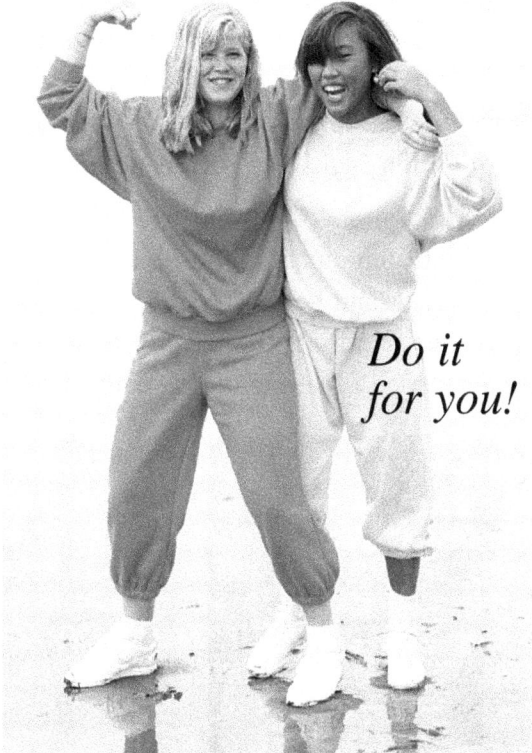

Do it for you!

Chapter 28: The roaring 20s:
Unfortunately, it can happen to you

Meet your inspiration

You will meet three amazing women from three different generations that have all mastered the art of changing their bodies. They are ordinary women facing the same, everyday challenges as all women. The only difference is that they were ready, had a plan, and followed through.

Although the stories are very different from each other, they prove that anyone really can transform her body regardless of any obstacles or any age. There are no excuses attached to any of these ladies, just results. So, whether you were heavy growing up, work full-time, had an eating disorder, have kids or any other situation you can possibly imagine, you will learn all the tricks and secrets to success—and be inspired.

I find it very gratifying and exciting that these women are looking to give back and help others by telling their stories as well as by incorporating fitness into their lives. Some have even have added fitness into their careers.

Meet Christina:
The early years

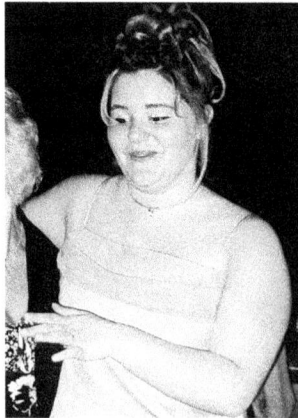

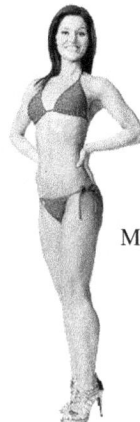

Meet Christina:
Today

The first time I met Christina was in 2011. She had a smile on her face filled with confidence. I would have never believed that she was ever overweight if it wasn't for her brother filling me in on her story.

Name: Christina Cores

Nickname: Cores

DOB 8/8/88

Hobbies: Kickboxing, motivational speaking, nutrition, bodybuilding

Favorite inspirational quote: "It doesn't happen by chance, it happens by choice"

In one word, how would others describe you? Tenacious

Height: 5'6

Weight before and after: My heaviest tracked weight was 240 lbs. My lowest weight was 118 lbs., but I typically fluctuate between 120 and 125 lbs.

Favorite music while working out: A mixture of pop, rock, hip hop, anything with a good beat to help me max out my work out

How long did it take you to achieve your body transformation?

I took my time with my weight loss and transformation because I wanted to achieve lasting results. I lost the weight in two years. My tone, strength, and physique have progressed over the last six years of maintaining the weight loss with proper nutrition and exercise.

Favorite cheat food: I love sweets! Cake, cookies, and chocolate are a weakness.

Tell us a little about yourself:

My weight loss made me feel so proud and good that I had the confidence to participate in a couple beauty pageants. To my surprise, I placed as a top ten finalist on the first one.

I had the great honor of being on the cover of "People" magazine's annual "Half Their Size" issue in January 2011. This led to appearances on the "Today" show, "Extra," "ET," and "Inside Edition." I've also been on the radio and in the newspaper. I've done motivational speaking; the most challenging place I spoke was in the very place I was bullied for my weight, my high school.

I'm now a certified personal trainer and am currently studying to be a nutrition coach. My future goals are to find a solid career in the fitness/nutrition field, and I'd love to do fitness modeling and more motivational speaking.

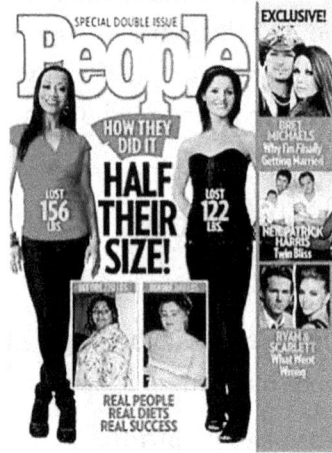

It seems like kids are so much more self-conscious about their bodies these days. Did you have any weight issues when you were younger? What do you blame it on? What made you make a change?

Actually, I had all my weight issues when I was younger. I started gaining weight at age 7, after my parents' divorce and all the changes that came with it. I come from an overweight family, so I naturally turned to food for comfort. I got bullied and picked on at school for being "fat," and I became an emotional eater who was steadily gaining weight each year.

School was so bad and hard for me that I constantly begged my mom to call me in sick. I couldn't deal with the looks, laughing, or crude comments. For gym class, I changed in the bathroom stalls because I was so ashamed and embarrassed for the girls to see my fat rolls and claw-like red and purple stretch marks on my stomach. I reached 240 pounds shortly after my dad's unexpected death, when I was 14 years old.

In high school, I would walk up a flight of stairs and be completely out of breath. I often ditched gym class because I couldn't keep up, and it was embarrassing. I couldn't cross my legs. I couldn't go shopping in the trendy teen stores.

What got you started in fitness?

I first turned to fitness to assist in my weight-loss goals. Initially, I hated working out. It was hard, took time, and was out of my comfort zone. However, I stuck with it because I was serious, committed, and was going to give it my all.

To my surprise, working out started becoming easier, and I was able to do things for longer periods of time. I could feel myself getting stronger while my body was getting smaller. I was proud of myself for every workout I completed, and it kept my nutrition on track because I refused to blow a workout that I just worked so hard for.

Were there any childhood eating habits that you wish would have been different?

Yes, growing up there were no restrictions. I was allowed to eat whatever I wanted, whenever I wanted, and as much as I wanted. My father's side of the family struggles with obesity, so naturally my dad enjoyed eating, and it became a way we bonded. I remember several times being woken up late at night to eat 1-pound burritos or to go get ice cream.

What's the biggest mistake you made when it came to trying to transform your body?

When I first started my transformation, I chose to go on a low-carb diet. It was popular at the time, and I was just learning about losing weight. The promise of quick weight loss intrigued me, so I jumped on the wagon and took it extremely seriously. I went as far as buying ketosis strips just to ensure that my body was in "fat-burning" mode.

Six months into this restrictive carb diet not only was it challenging and boring, but it started to negatively affect me physically. I felt dizzy and faint during my workouts. I came close to fainting a couple of times and had to sit down. This really scared me and was a true wake-up call. I thought I was doing the right thing because I was losing weight and working out, but my body was telling me otherwise.

This was a turning point in my transformation because I realized the importance of listening to your body. During my transformation, I made a commitment to myself to do it the "right" way to have lasting success. Everyone warned me about the danger of coming off a low-carb diet: "You'll gain the weight back plus more."

I was terrified to gain the weight back but didn't see it as scary as passing out in the middle of workouts. I continued my research and slowly and steadily brought good carbs back into my life. My weight loss was a little slower, but I was still losing, and now I had more energy for my workouts.

Research has shown that the next generation is the first one that will be outlived by their parents due to their obesity. What advice would you give to youngsters to keep their weight on the right track?

I would tell kids to be mindful of the choices they make because we each have only one body. The sooner we care about what we put into our bodies, the better life will become.

My advice to youngsters is that same peer pressure they're taught about in schools—to say no drugs and don't go along with it because everyone else is doing it—applies to what we feed our bodies. Whether its drugs or processed junk food, just because the cool kids think it's cool to eat candy and chips for lunch doesn't mean it's a good idea.

What problems could you foresee in the next decade as far as keeping your figure? How do you think you will deal with them?

I've worked with many middle-aged women and their weight-loss goals. I already have a preview of what to expect as I age. I know my metabolism will change as I age, and I know that what I do now for my fitness, nutrition, and health will impact the future.

I'm concerned about when I decide to have children. It's going to be hard for me psychologically to accept the weight gain. Of course, I will have my child's best interest in mind, but it is something I see myself struggling with. I have high hopes and goals to be an active, healthy pregnant chic. I've promised myself to not let pregnancy be an excuse to eat junk and be lazy.

Do you think the habits you have recently adopted will easily follow you for the rest of your life?

I absolutely agree that that these habits will follow me the rest of my life because I see it as a lifestyle change, and I've kept the weight off for more than 6 years. I don't think it "easily" follows me. My eyes may be bigger than my stomach from time to time, but it's keeping my mind strong that keeps me on track.

There is so much misinformation out there about what to eat and what not to eat. What type of nutrition plan do you currently follow (include an example day with beverages)?

My eating program was focused on nutrition, portion control, and swapping bad choices with better choices.

I try to stay away from fried foods, processed foods, and fast foods. I also make a point not to drink my calories. I avoid juices and high-caloric, high-sugar drinks.

I always read labels and sometimes still log my food. My diet largely consists of oatmeal, eggs, lean proteins such as chicken, nuts, yogurt, fruits, veggies, brown rice, protein shakes, and protein bars. I drink lots of water.

I found that watching sodium can be useful, and it's something that so many people overlook. I got so good at reading labels and knowing how many calories something was that, once I had lost the weight, many times I could keep track of things in my head. Numbers are very important in the beginning and during the journey, but I discovered that once I hit my weight loss goals, I tried really listening to my body.

Example day:

Breakfast: Coffee; oatmeal with half sliced banana and walnuts; hard-boiled egg; water

Snack protein shake or bar

 Lunch: Vitamin water; lower-sodium, no-nitrates-or-added-hormones turkey wrap with lettuce, tomato, cucumber, three-cheese pepper hummus instead of mayo; and a yogurt

Snack water, apple with peanut butter

Dinner: diet soda; boneless, skinless grilled chicken breast; asparagus tossed in a little olive oil; brown rice

What workout program seems to keep your body looking its best these days? (give example of a typical workout or what videos do you do)

I first started with a workout video. Within a few weeks, I joined a women's-only club that was a combination of strength training and cardio in a circuit fashion. The workout was 30 minutes three times a week. I used this regimen for quite a while until I joined a co-ed gym that had all the equipment I could ever dream of.

I purposely chose to go to the gym during non-peak times so

I'd feel more comfortable and not look silly while I figured out how to use the machines. I'd use the treadmill and stair master for cardio. I used the weighted machines and dumb-bells. The stability ball became my best friend for ab work-outs. I didn't have a set program; it was more about the variety.

On days when I felt less motivated, I'd go to a group fitness class, which helped me push myself harder. I would do some type of cardio with every workout. As I got stronger and more toned and defined, I would have a leg day, arm day, back, etc. so I'd really develop muscular strength.

Do you think it's possible to transform your body without going to a gym?

Yes, I believe you can transform your body without going to the gym. Gyms aren't for everyone. It's about finding something you like and, most importantly, will do! Gyms are filled with the tools, education, and help to achieve your dream body, so I do encourage them. Transformations require commitment and dedication not necessarily a gym membership.

What's your workout philosophy?

Working out is preventative medication and the greatest stress reliever! I constantly hear of younger and younger people going on blood pressure pills, getting diagnosed with diabetes, and so on. The combination of nutrition and work-ing out not only will change how you look on the outside but does wonders for long-term health. My philosophy is the days you really don't want to work out are the most impor-tant days to do the workout. You're one workout away from a good mood and better health.

How many hours per week do you work out?

It varies at different times of the year. I aim for 6 to 8 hours a week but do a minimum of 3 hours a week.

Have you fallen off the wagon and gained weight back? If so, what got you off track, and how did you deal with it to get yourself back on track?

I'm human not an angel. I think we all go through times when we find ourselves slacking nutritionally and physically. I feel it in my clothes, energy level, and my mood when I "fall off" the wagon. The most I've gained is 8 pounds, but I hate the way I feel when I'm off track.

What made you make fitness part of your career?

When I started my transformation, I didn't believe in myself. I didn't believe I'd lose the weight or keep it off. However, once I did, I discovered confidence, pride, and passion. I found that fitness and nutrition, the things that used to be my enemies were my new best friends. I made the jump because I wanted to help others believe in themselves.

Finding motivation is the toughest thing to get people going. What motivates you to consistently stay on track?

I constantly read articles and magazines related to fitness/nutrition. I read success stories and make inspiration boards.

What's your favorite healthy recipe?

Oven-baked chicken fajitas

Below are excuses that I hear most from women as to why they can't change their bodies. How would you respond to any one of them that stand out to you?

Don't have the time

I don't feel like it

My back hurts

I'm too tired

I'm too busy

My kids take up my time

Exercise is boring

I don't have the motivation

My alarm didn't go off this morning

I'm too old to start a program

I can't afford to go to a gym

I don't have any equipment

I don't know what to do

My dog ate my workout clothes

I always hear people say they don't have time to change their bodies between jobs, children, etc. All I hear is excuse after excuse. You have to make the time for the things that matter most to you. If you have time for television and Facebook, you have time for exercise! It may take some creativity fitting fitness into a busy schedule, but it can and should be done. Every little bit of effort you put towards exercise counts and will make you feel better than ever.

Are there any other comments you would like to share with those trying to transform their bodies that may help them reach their dream body?

Do this for yourself, and pay no attention to those around who doubt you. Don't give up ever! It does take time. It's very challenging but it's absolutely WORTH IT! Don't beat yourself up for the bad days or slack days just don't let them become bad weeks!

When you hit the dreaded plateau, remember to focus on how far you've come, not how far you have to go. Learn to listen to your body and focus on becoming the best version of yourself rather than comparing yourself to others.

Chapter 29: **The roaring 30s:**
Who said I can't do this?

Meet Mary: A detail orientated spitfire

Although some women are well established in life by the time they hit 30, many women are just starting out. This is typically a time of big changes, as careers are taking off and children are entering their lives with all sorts of commotion. This decade can bring on a whirlwind of change. Change, good or bad, is always hard to deal with.

When I met Mary, she was a sweet girl who I thought had her whole fitness plan figured out. This is sometimes the problem with trainers. When clients seem like they know what they are talking about, we tend to leave them alone.

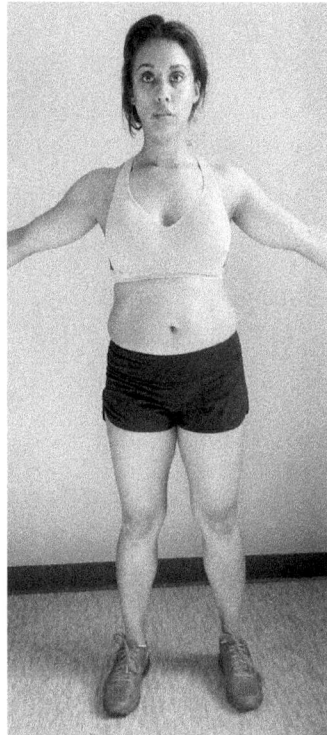

Mary had an OK understanding of working harder but not necessarily smarter. She would see a workout on the internet or in a magazine and think that it would work for anyone, including her. We actually learned from each other what worked best for her body when it came to transforming it.

Mary built muscle very quickly with heavier weights, and everyone told her that is what she needed to do to change her body.

We changed that: Mary's biggest need was her eating plan. She was lost when it came to what to eat and when. Take a look at how Mary has made fitness a priority in her life, even with two little kids keeping her busy.

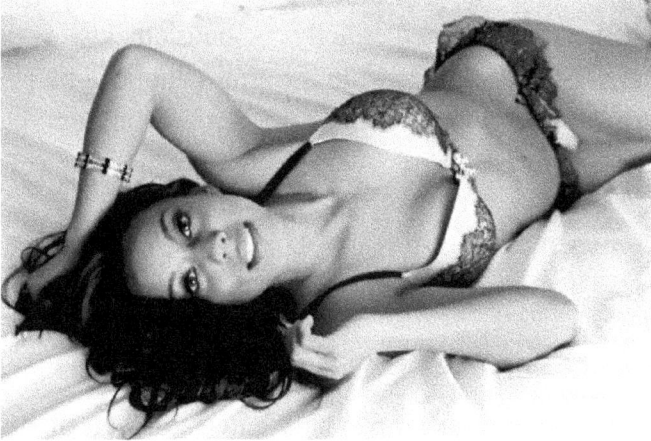

Name: Mary Mandujano

Age: 32

Hobbies: Movie junkie, kickboxing, martial arts, sprint-distance triathlons and community service projects

Favorite quote: "We must always change, renew, rejuvenate ourselves, otherwise we harden and set in our ways." ~ Johann Wolfgang Von Goethe

In one word, how would others describe you?
Compassionate

Height? 5'4 + ½ "
Weight? 124.8 lbs
Body Fat? 13.1%
Heaviest Weight? 150
Highest Body Fat? 24.5%

How long did it take you to achieve your body transformation? 10 weeks

Favorite food: Chick-Fil-A

Favorite body part(s) to train? Why?

Arms/Shoulders. My upper body responds quickly to weight training. Muscle definition in the arms is noticed by people right away and normally gives the impression that you hit the gym on a regular basis.

Most frustrating part(s) of your body to slim down or tame? Thighs and triceps

Toughest health/fitness challenge you had to tackle?

Discipline in packing up meals and eating clean during those lengthy holiday seasons that fall back-to-back like Thanksgiving-Christmas-New Years.

Tell us a little about yourself.

I am Hispanic, born and raised in Wisconsin, and have six older siblings. I graduated from Southwestern University in Texas with a B.S. in international business. I worked in human resources at S.C. Johnson, Case New Holland, and GE Healthcare. I now co-own a translation company for criminal and immigration law.

I have two toddler boys who keep me on my toes and demand of lot of my time and energy. To stay sane between part-time work and kids, the gym has become my stress-relieving sanctuary.

Last year, I signed on with GlobalOne LLC, a modeling agency in Los Angeles. This hobby has been a huge motivation for me, but it has also put different fitness challenges in my path. Fortunately, I've had a great coach to help me with diet plans and workout programs to achieve the results required for different photo shoots.

What got you started in fitness?

From elementary school through college, I was on sports teams. In my last two years of college, I had ankle ligament reconstruction surgery and my class load called for more study time. The little free time that was left went to basic gym workouts and going to movies.

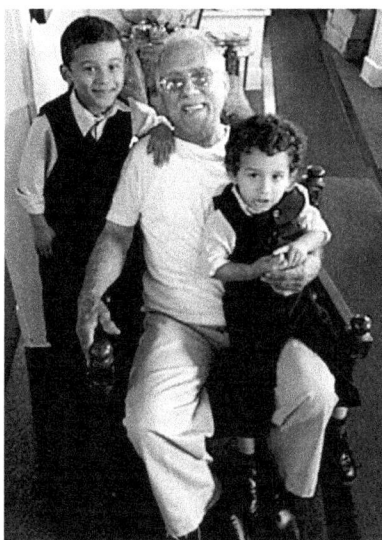

Mary's father and children

While in college, two significant things helped me define "fitness" and convicted me of its importance: my dad had heart bypass surgery in his 60s, and I read T. Colin Campbell's book "The China Study."

After surgery, my dad was told to change his eating habits and add exercise to his daily routine. Coming home from the hospital, he literally cleared out the refrigerator and changed his lifestyle.

My dad has become my role model because such discipline

is not easy to maintain. Now 76, he is self-confident, full of energy and does military exercises (using only body weight) to stay fit. He babysits my toddlers and plays with them from the time they arrive until the time they leave. It's dynamic to see how nutrition and exercise magnify a person's vitality and keep his or her body going.

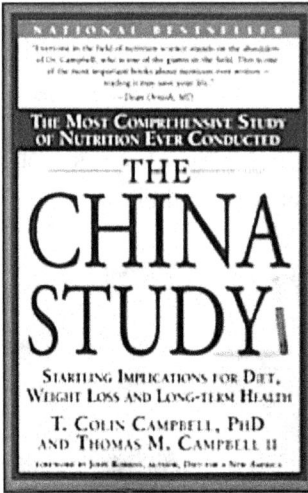

In 2003, I read "The China Study." Campbell is a nutritional scientist at Cornell University. The "New York Times" recognizes the book as the "Grand Prix of epidemiology" and the "most comprehensive study ever undertaken of the relationship between diet and the risk of developing disease."

It clarifies the misperceptions that have shaped our way of thinking and eating as a nation. If you want to get deep about nutrition, get your hands on a copy of this book! Don't like to read thick books? See a condensed version on DVD, "Forks over Knives," a documentary that will inspire you to eat well. You will see things in a much different perspective and will appreciate health on a greater scale.

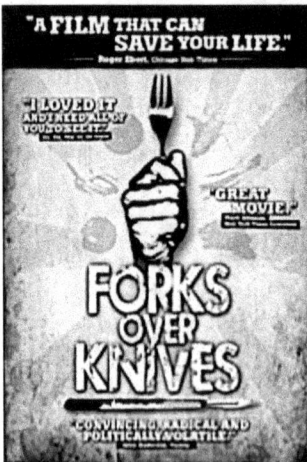

Did you ever struggle with your weight when you were younger?

As a child and throughout my teenage years, I was very slender. I had a difficult time gaining weight despite what and how much I ate. I badly wanted my body to "fill out" and get the curves I expected to develop, especially as a Hispanic female.

It wasn't until college, when I got into soccer, that I finally developed an athletic body and reached 130 pounds. After college, throughout my career, and after my first pregnancy, I maintained a weight of 135 pounds. It wasn't until after my second pregnancy when I struggled at 150 pounds.

You had two kids as you entered your 30s. How did this affect your body, and how did you overcome this?

Both of my pregnancies were a breeze; the weight came off quickly, and nursing helped keep it off. I was back at 135 pounds but with a saggy stomach from stretched skin. Nonetheless, I was looking forward to repeating the routine I had developed after my first baby – hitting the gym and keeping up with good eating habits. To my frustration, however, this second time around wasn't so smooth.

Between a 16-month-old and his newborn brother, I had no free time. Throughout the week, I ate anything that was quick and convenient. Because I was always rushing, my meals were quick and small, but it didn't take much of eating the wrong kind of things to pack on the weight.

Friends and family saw my time-management struggle but, instead of offering to babysit so that I could go to the gym, they brought me homemade dishes (delicious but unhealthy) and filled my pantry with bread, tortillas, cookies, chips and other snacks.

A month went by, and I stepped on the scale: 150 pounds?! My leniency had cost me 15 pounds in only four weeks. I got depressed, and I got angry.

A few weeks into the new schedule, I was sweating my butt off during workouts and I was back to eating healthy (so I thought) but my body wasn't responding the same way. I exhausted my ideas and finally turned to the best personal trainer at my gym for help. I received general nutrition guidance, 1-on-1 personal training sessions twice a week, and body assessments on a regular basis to track progress.

For the nutrition piece, my trainer took out "reds" (beef and pork), "whites" (pasta/potatoes/breads/white rice/processed-flour items), and recommended I load my meals with vegetables. I ate limited amounts of turkey, chicken and fish. During this same time period, I was attending the "Complete Health Improvement Program" (CHIP), which educates the community on health, diet and disease.

Because I was not given a calorie-count diet by my trainer, I decided to test the CHIP program. I put my trainer's nutrition list together with CHIP's three-meals-per-day plan. At the end of five weeks, my body fat had melted from 24% to 18%.

After that, I set aside personal training but attended free group exercise classes and maintained the basic diet. Not much later, progress came to a sudden halt; there was no more weight loss. I felt as if I had hit a brick wall and could not pinpoint what was keeping me from advancing. I convinced myself that I had plateaued.

Surprisingly, that same year, I received an offer to join GlobalOne. I knew more bodywork maintenance was needed. I got worried, and Rob Boyce offered help. He provided strict, customized diets; workout programs; food journals; and assessment tracking.

Under his rules, I was to eat five or six times a day, with meals divided into a carbs/proteins/fats ratio and calorie limit. The first three weeks were great, and then the holidays came. It became difficult to stick with the meal plan, so I let myself fail!

To start the New Year on a clean slate, I went back to Rob for round two. This time, I was mentally ready. Within weeks of following his program, I transformed my body from a stubborn 18% body fat down to 13% body fat.

There are three things worth considering to overcome obstacles as I did:

(1) Workouts will be a waste of time if you don't fully understand and apply the 80/20 concept (80% of your efforts account for diet and 20% for exercise). You may think you are eating healthy when, in reality, your "definition" may have a few loopholes. The fact that I didn't eat fast food or processed snacks led me to believe that I was eating healthy, so I expected my body to respond as it did after my first pregnancy. Looking back, my metabolism had slowed down.

(2) With the help of a trainer, set a reasonable deadline to reach your goal, and live up to it. Do not base your success solely on weight loss; have frequent body-fat assessments to

measure body-fat reduction to detect real progress.

(3) As you age, have children, or acquire injuries, accept the fact that these things will cause your body to change, slow down and/or respond differently. They will affect things such as metabolism, energy, recovery rate, CNS response, flexibility, physical competence, etc. Don't give up hope. There are ways of working around and through these obstacles, but you must seek guidance and be willing to work harder for results.

Did you have any obstacles in your 20s that may have set you up for failure or any good habits that set you up for success as you entered your 30s?

In my 20s, I ate whatever I wanted, however much I wanted, whenever I wanted. This habit became an obstacle for me after my second pregnancy and as I entered my 30s.

I had to reprogram my way of eating based on how my body changed, my metabolism, and its physical response. Attention to diet and discipline becomes key. Replacing bad habits with good ones made the transition easier for me. Taking it steps at a time helped establish the new routine into a consistent one.

Being a mother of two and working odd/long hours, how do you make sure you get your workouts in to maintain or improve your body?

I established specific workout times, length of workouts, and number of days of the week to exercise. I wrote the phrase "workout 8 a.m." every Monday, Wednesday and Friday on my wall calendar so that I could mentally record that schedule. I had two alarms set—one at 7 a.m. and the second at 7:15 a.m. in case I failed to wake up. I also packed up my workout clothes into my gym bag the night prior and set it by the door with my water bottle and purse so it was easy to just grab-and-go.

I went as far as to posting a picture of a model whose body composition was close to what I wanted on my bathroom mirror. It motivated me to get going in the mornings and served as a reminder as to why I was waking up early to exercise. On those designated mornings, at exactly 7:30 a.m., I would leave to the gym, start my workouts at 8 a.m. and be in the women's locker room ready to shower by 9:15 a.m. Knowing myself, this was the only way to make things happen.

Time seems to be an obstacle or excuse for many working women with kids. What advice would you have for them to be successful in changing their bodies and "making" time?

By nature, every mother has the ability to play many roles and still function well on a daily basis; God just made us that way. There comes a point, however, when working mothers, and stay-at-home moms alike, need to set aside time to release physically and re-energize psychologically. Otherwise we'll find ourselves pulling our hair out and going crazy.

Time is a luxury, yes, but putting priority to what you hold dear to your heart will determine whether it gets done or tossed away. Rather than saying, "How can I exercise if I don't have time?" say, "How am I going to make this work?"

If you spend most of your time at work, partner with a co-worker to bring healthy lunches or take brisk walks during lunch. If you can't go to the gym because you don't have a sitter or don't like taking your kids to the gym's daycare, then invest your money in a cardio machine to use at home. Exercise equipment doesn't have to be new; you can find deals on websites like Craigslist and Ebay.

Once you purchase equipment, set up your home gym where part of the room will be "child friendly." Assuming your children are quite young and semi-dependent, you'll want to keep an eye on them while exercising but have them be distracted enough to allow you to workout. Drag some toys into that section of the room for them to play with or have a snack table ready to satisfy their appetite while they watch a movie on your laptop. My boys love toy trains, so I bought a used train table with a large train set and accessories. It has kept them occupied for up to an hour, giving me freedom to exercise.

Depending on your kids' ages, be realistic and be reasonable; tailor your workout length to what your children can handle on their own. Expect interruptions while you're trying to establish the routine, but be consistent with your workout schedule so your children can get into the same routine.

If you're still finding it difficult making time to exercise or you're really just stuck at home, have a personal trainer come to you instead. This alternative may help you feel more obligated to meet your appointments and make you more receptive to reforming your habits. If you feel you can't afford "at-home" personal training, perhaps you can get a "buddy rate." Find a friend, maybe one who also has children, and you'll kill two birds with one stone: playmates for your kids and a motivational workout buddy to train with.

Don't waste your money on fast food because it's the convenient thing to do for the sake of time; to avoid frustration from having to cook every day, set aside one day of the week to make your own healthy microwavable lunches and dinners. Yes, it will require a few hours for preparation, cooking, packaging, and cleaning a messy kitchen, but it saves you the hustle and bustle throughout the week!

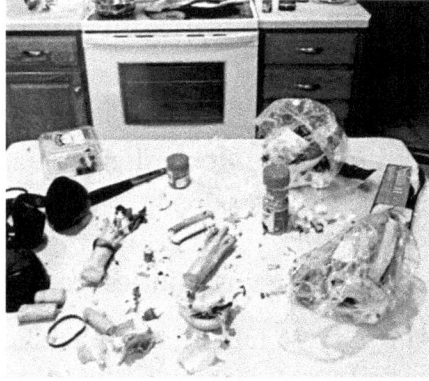

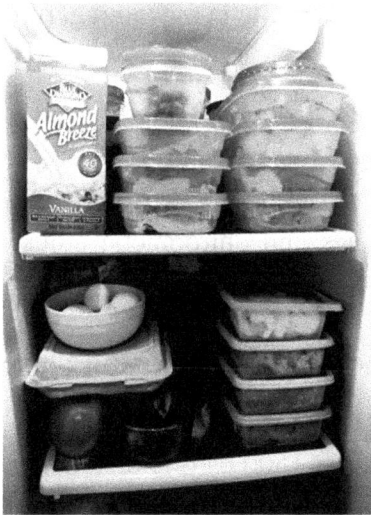

Put together your meals for the week, and put them in food containers so you can just reach into the refrigerator to "heat-and-eat" or "take-and-go."

Be creative, be patient, share and exchange ideas with your friends, and you will ultimately find a method that will work for you.

How have your workouts changed over the last ten years?

I was on corporate athletic sports teams at SC Johnson. A few years later, when I transferred to GE Healthcare, I did group exercise classes and then joined corporate teams who competed in local triathlons. Triathlon training required numerous hours of swimming, running and cycling throughout the week.

After I had my boys, I switched to basic gym workouts, group exercise classes and kickboxing. Most recently, I have been following Rob's strength-training exercises to acquire muscle and a lean body.

Do you have any injuries from when you were younger?

At age six, I fell off an 8-foot slide and landed on my tailbone. I didn't feel the effects of the injury until high school, when I became heavily involved in sports and martial arts. During college, I had ankle ligament reconstruction surgery. To this day, my ankle still gives out while I am walking, running or jumping.

I try to rotate between different types of exercises, such as weight training, kickboxing, cardio and group exercise classes, because each type gives your body a different experience. I have monthly massages and chiropractic adjustments to keep my body aligned.

What is your typical eating program? How does it differ from what you used to eat?

My typical day consists of a 1,200-1500 calorie diet, eating five to six times a day.

The menu consists of: Ezekiel bread, oats, rice cakes, brown rice, jasmine rice, quinoa, black beans, egg whites, almond milk, almond butter, apples, blueberries, raspberries, and cherries. Meats consist of tuna, tilapia, salmon, lean turkey. The main vegetables are asparagus, cauliflower, broccoli, spinach leaves, sweet potatoes, and hummus. For condiments, I use grapeseed oil and McCormick seasonings (lightly used). I drink four or more 32oz. bottles of water throughout the day for hydration, digestion and weight loss.

Compared to how I used to eat, I now consume fewer carbs, more protein, no breads, no soups, no salt, no butter, no dairy products (except eggs) and a calorie-count limit for each meal.

What's your favorite healthy recipe?

Lemon-pepper salmon brushed with grapeseed oil, topped with sliced almonds, and a side of asparagus.

How many days per week do you work out?

I workout 4 to 5 times a week for 60 minutes.

What workout program seems to work best for you?

Lighter weights work best for me as my body builds muscle fairly quickly, and I get bulky with the typical 8 to 12 reps of heavier weights. This is why it is so important not to follow a cookie-cutter approach to your program. You have to do what works best for you.

Can you give examples of some workouts you do?

Trainers always told me to do heavy weights to build muscle but Rob and I found that, with my shorter stature, I gain muscle pretty quickly in my legs. So we did lighter weights in the 15+ rep range for my legs and sculpted my upper body with heavier weights in the 8 to 12 repetition range.

I alternate between upper and lower body workouts, and my cardio workouts were initially done on the elliptical machine. My cardio workouts followed the strength routines 4 days per week.

In the first few weeks, I kept my heart rate at a steady level of 145 beats per minutes for 30 minutes. During weeks 4 to 8, I did interval training on the elliptical machine: 1 minute at 125 bpm and one minute at 155 for a total of 20 minutes.

For the last 2 weeks, I did two cardio workouts per day, one in the morning and one in the evening. I kept the same interval program but tried to stay in the 155 bpm range for 2 minutes at a time.

What motivates you to keep going?

My father—he's made me a full believer in healthy living. My dad stays dedicated to a clean diet and exercise.

My boys—I hope to live a long, healthy life so that I can see my boys grow up. I want to be an active and supportive parent in

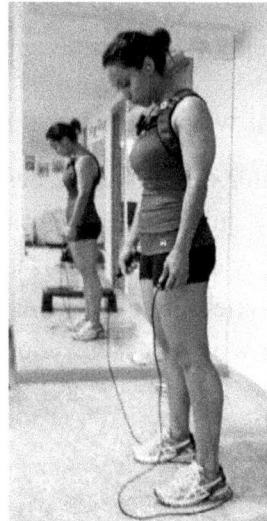

activities, events and sports that they will take interest in. My desire is that they will value healthy living by seeing their grandpa and their mom as strong examples.

Other women—I am motivated to be an inspiration to females, particularly in the Hispanic culture. Fitness and healthy eating is uncommon to this ethnicity. Traditional high-in-fat food dishes and style of eating has jeopardized younger generations into early stages of obesity.

Modeling—This has been an exciting hobby for me. It calls for different demands and physique expectations for every photo shoot.

How would you respond to these excuses that I hear most often?

I don't have the time. I'm too busy.

Make time for exercise just as you do for work, to eat, and to go to the bathroom.

I don't feel like it.

Exercise when you least feel like it. Chances are you're feeling tired, stressed or lazy. Exercise is a great way to relieve stress, regain energy and build up your immune system.

I'm too tired.

If you're feeling tired on a regular basis, you may not be eating right or enough to replenish the energy you depleted from your day. You also may have a deficiency that needs to be met; take a whole-food multivitamin.

My kids take up my time.

Almost every gym offers daycare, so you have no excuse there. If you dislike the daycare, then workout from home. Invest your money in a few basic workout items like a stability ball, medicine ball, band, and dumbbells. Then, go online and search "workout videos."

Exercise is boring, and I don't have the motivation.

Find a friend, neighbor or co-worker to be your exercise buddy and set times to meet each week so that you feel obligated and accountable to follow through with the plan. If your exercise buddy fails to meet with you on a regular basis, go to plan B. Consider joining a group exercise class at your gym or a boot camp that will expose you to a larger group of people where encouragement and push will come at you from all directions.

Is there any other advice you would give to ladies entering their 30s looking to transform their bodies?

Patience and persistence is the name of the game. Your "can-do" attitude will take you places you never imagined. And yes, it's a mental game. On your path to wellness, what goes on inside your head is just as important as the food you eat and the exercise you complete. What you believe influences what you will accomplish.

Don't get frustrated with yourself and give up; allow room for trial and error at the beginning of your transformation journey. Any time you catch yourself thinking "I can't," replace the thought with, "I can if I break it down into doable steps."

If you need someone to push you, invest your money and time in a trainer for a solid two months. After some time, you will become acquainted with your body and understand how it responds to certain food plans and exercise programs. When you start to notice that your clothes are looser and people are noticing and complimenting your transformation, this will flip your motivation switch, helping you stay on your wellness program.

Track your progress with a fitness tracker to understand your advancement by the numbers. This will not only motivate you but will also point out any stubborn body sections that may need more attention. Numerous studies show that self-efficacy is one of the most important determining factors in whether someone maintains a new habit and sticks with it.

Log your meals in a food journal to help track how any calories you are consuming. It is very easy to overeat and very easy to underestimate the amount of calories in a food item. Read your food labels carefully so you don't overlook the serving size in correlation to the calorie amount.

Drinking a lot of water will do wonders for your body; eight glasses a day is the minimum you should have. Keep in mind that while you are on a specific meal plan or special diet, you may have to temporarily eliminate "girls' night out" from your calendar or limit hangouts with friends who love to drink and eat out at restaurants and bars. If you can handle the pressure and resist temptation, carry on!

To stay sane, allow yourself one cheat meal per week, but don't go overboard; stay within a calorie limit, and choose an entrée wisely. From personal experience, because I wanted to maintain a social lifestyle, I would eat my specific meal plan before hanging out with family or friends. While they were ordering a high-in-fat, loaded-calorie entrée at the restaurant, I could make a wiser decision and select a low-calorie grilled chicken salad (without dressing) or a tilapia-vegetable plate. Because I had already eaten my specific meal two hours prior, it became much easier to dodge the emotional "urge-to-splurge" mood.

If you have a fast-paced life and need to find another alternative to eating well throughout your day, carry protein or food bars in your purse or put a snack pack together and carry it in your car.

My snack pack included: *A copy of my meal plan*

One scoop of IsoPure Protein powder in a cylinder tupperware,

One scoop of Advocare's Post Workout Recovery Protein powder in a cylinder tupperware,

Lean Body Meal Replacement packet,

QuestBar Protein Bar,

Lean Body Protein bar,

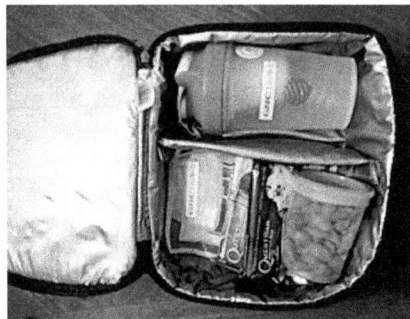

Cup of almonds,

My Vitamin case contained: 1 whole-food vitamin, 3 capsules Nature's Sunshine Proactazyme Plus (to aid digestion), 1 gel capsule Advocare OmegaPlex (fish oil) and 3 capsules Advocare Catalyst (Amino Acid)

Used as substitutes:

Almond butter, travel-size spoon & knife

2 Rice cakes in glass tupperware

5 oz canned tuna & mini can opener

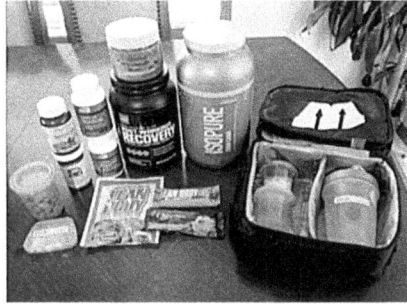

I also posted photos on my bathroom mirror and refrigerator door. I wanted positive reminders to help me stay focused and not veer from my meal plan. One read: "Healthy eating and exercise shows that you control your body, don't let it control you." Fitness magazines on the table where I sit down to eat also help me stay on track.

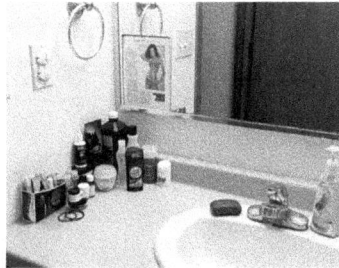

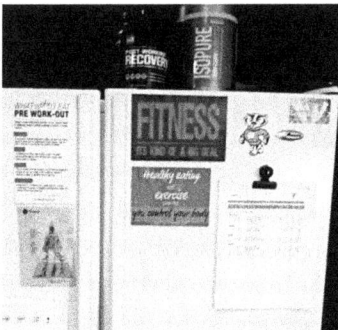

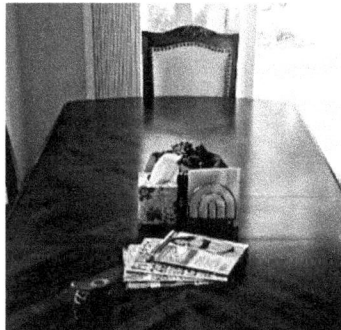

Finally, no one shows up at the gym every day feeling motivated and pumped. Some days you wonder how and why you got to the gym because you're not in fire-mode. I posted signs ad photos on my locker door and would contemplate them while changing into my workout clothes.

Remember, training starts in the brain.

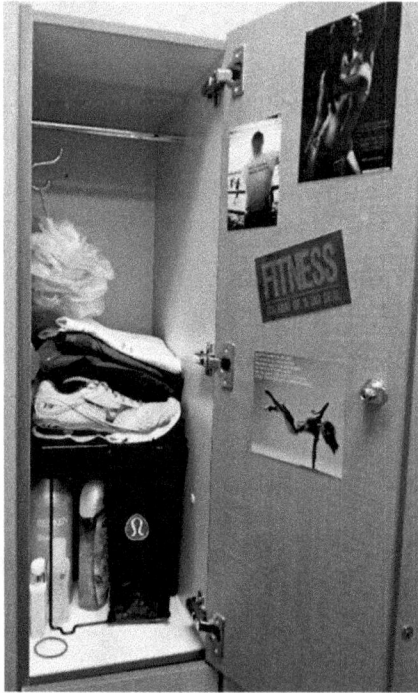

Chapter 30:   The big 4-0:
Looking better than a 20 year old feels pretty good

Could the 40s be the new 20s?

Meet Cheryl: *She will never be known as a quitter*

I don't think Cheryl knew what a fruit or vegetable tasted like and pretty much stayed thin. She worked out very hard and probably too much. So, how could she possibly change her body when she was 5'6" and 125 pounds at age 46?

Many people would tell her, "You don't need to work out, you look great." But she had a goal in her own mind that she set out to achieve. She took it to the next level and made time even though she had three teenage kids, took care of the house, worked 40-plus hours per week, had two dogs, and was studying for a test she was passionate about. (By the way, by the time this book was completed, she passed her test and is currently a certified personal trainer through the NASM CPT.)

She still managed to train her body to be better looking than 90% of 20 year olds. She took first place in a fitness figure competition. It wasn't all perfect, though; Cheryl battled an eating disorder early on in her life.

I can't tell you how many women have stepped in my office at age 40 and blamed their poor fitness on hitting this magic number. They would suggest that, when they hit 40, inevitably their body was not going to be the same as when it was 20, nor would they want it to be. I always found this a bit strange. Why wouldn't you want to be in the best shape of your life and look your best regardless of your age? I have come to realize that these comments are simply excuses before they even start their plan.

109

When you hit 40, you are engrained in your ways, and it is very difficult to change. So it's time to open your mind and see how Cheryl did it.

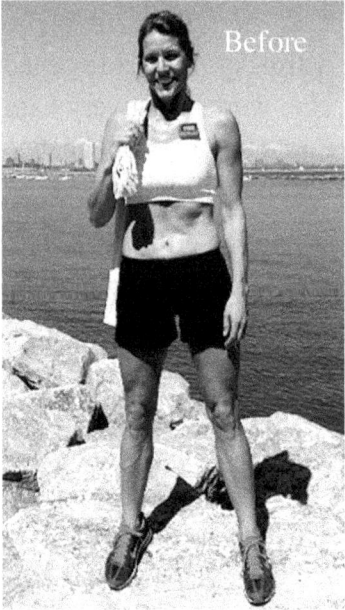

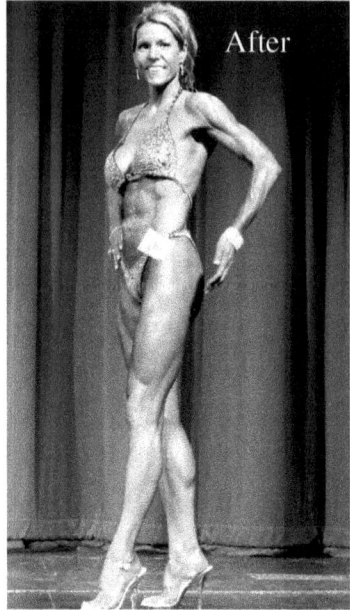

Name: Cheryl

Nicknames: Cracker, C-dog and Lil Bit

Age: 46

Hobbies: baking, reading, home improvement projects, crafts and shopping

Favorite Quote: "Our lives are not determined by what happens to us, but by how we react to what happens; not by what life brings to us, but by the attitude we bring to life. A positive attitude causes a chain reaction of positive thoughts, events and outcomes. It is a catalyst... a spark that creates extraordinary results."

In one word, how would others describe you: Driven

Favorite Foods: Chipotle, Dominos, Quest Bars and Peanut Butter (now almond butter)

Height: 5' 6-1/2"

Beginning Weight: 122.8 3/2013

Beginning Body Fat: 17.4% 3/2013

Final Weight: 119 5/2013

Final Body Fat: 8% 5/2013

Competition Body Transformation: 11 weeks

Tell us a little about yourself:

I am your typical 46 year old, energetic mom of boys ages 17, 19, and 21.

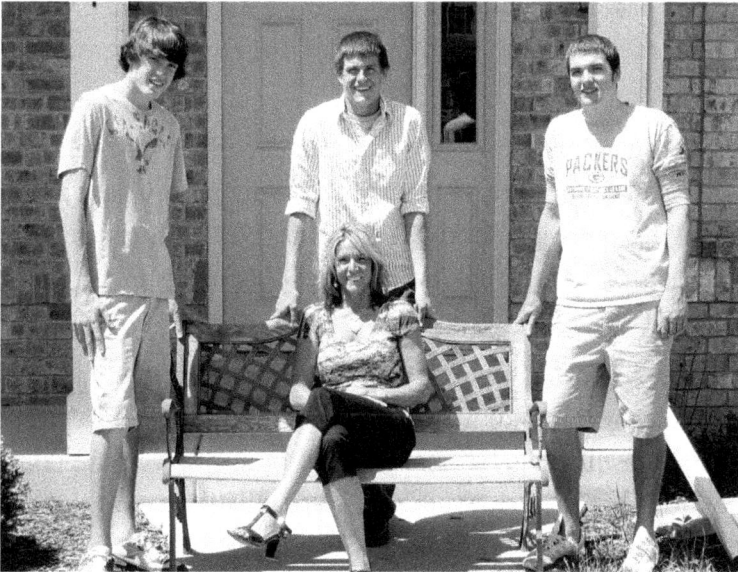

Like most women, I am constantly searching to find that perfect balance between children, family, friends, careers, household responsibilities, extracurricular activities, social life, spiritual life, health and fitness and sleep (with sleep getting the smallest piece of the pie).

Speaking of pie, one of my favorite hobbies is baking. Like working out, baking is a stress reliever for me. Fortunately, I don't indulge too much in the goodies but do my best to keep everything in moderation.

I grew up in Niagara, a small town in northern Wisconsin, where I lived with my parents, two older brothers and my older sister; I loved being the baby. I was very active in high school athletics (basketball, volleyball, track) and also participated in dance (tap and jazz) for 9 years. I became involved in fitness my first summer out of high school, when I got a job with a small fitness center. I quickly developed a passion for fitness that continued into college, where I became an aerobics instructor for the University of Wisconsin-Whitewater.

While fitness was not part of my career path, it has remained a constant in my life. I have built on my on my passion by receiving my BeachBody Turbo Kick certification, becoming a boot-camp instructor, and obtaining my NASM Personal Training Certification.

I have competed in many 5K and 10k races, triathlons, obstacles races, and, my most recent accomplishment (May 2013) was placing 1st, 2nd and 4th in my first figure competition. I feel a great sense of accomplishment in reaching my health and fitness goals but feel an even greater sense of accomplishment when I can help others reach their goals.

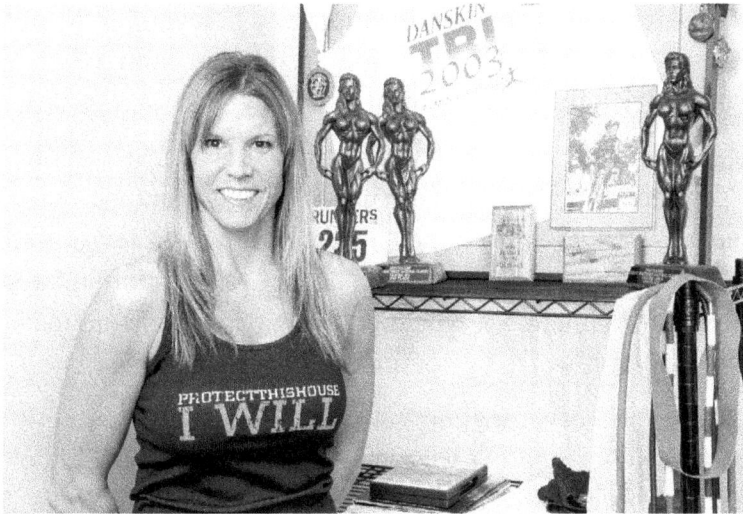

A lot of women say that when they hit 40 their metabolism slows, which is the reason they carry extra weight. What are your thoughts on this statement?

Research seems to have some pretty solid evidence to indicate that women put on weight after the age of 40 due to a slower metabolism, so I guess I won't waste my time arguing science; however, we need place blame where blame is due. Weight gain and being out of shape are more due to accepting slow metabolism as a way of life, as something inevitable. A slow metabolism becomes an easy excuse, a scapegoat.

Our bodies function differently at various stages of our life, and we have to understand these changes and adapt our lifestyles. My first defense against this demon was hitting the weights and, secondly, cleaning up my diet. To my surprise, eating clean was much more enjoyable and easier than I thought.

There is a bigger concern for injuries when you hit 40 and above. Have you had any major injuries, and what is your advice for keeping injuries at bay?

Despite many years of intense working out, I have had only a few minor injuries, and nothing that has taken me out of the game for too long. I had an issue with my knee as well as my lower back. In both cases, I tried to work through the discomfort thinking it would go away on its own and made the condition worse by continuing to workout.

After weeks of struggling with a lower back issue and not being able to bend over and put my socks on, I finally took Rob's advice and went to see a chiropractor. Within days, I was feeling a drastic improvement and, within a week, was almost back to my same workout intensity. I still continue to go for maintenance and feel it has been the key to keeping me injury free for the most part.

In both cases, my discomfort was the result of tight muscles. My advice is to incorporate a proper warm up and cool down with every workout. Myofascial release (foam roller) therapy worked wonders for improving my flexibility, function and performance.

Also, don't be afraid to seek medical attention. The longer you go without treatment, the more damage you can do. And most importantly, listen to your body.

The biggest excuse I hear from women is that they don't have time. How would you respond to that excuse?

That excuse is exactly that, an excuse. My response to that comment, as well as the hundreds of other excuses I have heard is, "There are excuses and there are results, never both."

Exercise needs to be scheduled into your calendar just like any other important thing in your life. For me, the best way to ensure I get my workout in is to exercise at 4:30 a.m., before I go to work, before anyone in the house is up, before the day starts getting hectic, and before life can get in the way. The only excuse I am left with is not being able to get my butt out of bed.

Also, keep in mind that you don't need an hour to get an effective workout. HIIT (High Intensity Interval Training) workouts are some of my favorite, and, in 10 to 20 minutes, you can get in a great, fat-burning workout. Any workout (even if it is only 10 minutes) is better than no workout at all.

The odds are almost every woman in her 40s has tried some quick-fix diet to change her body. Is there a secret diet they should know about?

Keep it simple: Burn more calories than you consume.

Some women say exercise is not fun. What would you tell them that would change their minds about exercise or motivate them?

I've always enjoyed working out, so I'm fortunate that I haven't had to overcome this barrier so many women face.

Yes, some days I'm just not feeling it, and I need to dig deep for motivation. I'm not sure if it is the actual physical part of working out that I enjoy so much or the psychological benefits I reap from a great workout. I think the key is variety and finding something that's fun for you.

If you enjoy dancing, try Zumba. If you're competitive, maybe a team activity is your thing, and, if you like working out with others, maybe a group fitness class would motivate you. Try a variety of options, and figure out what you enjoy so that it is easier to stay committed. Blasting good music seems to motivate me and makes my workouts more fun. If the treadmill, elliptical or stationary bike are boring to you, try watching your favorite show while on them.

When I'm faced with a real challenge or goal, I have used a reward system as a fun way to stay motivated.

For example, put aside a dollar every time you workout. When you reach $100, treat yourself.

Finding a workout buddy is another popular way to make working out more enjoyable and tends to keep people accountable. You might not feel like getting out of bed to get to class, but the guilt of coming up with an excuse and cancelling on your friend is even harder to do. If you don't have the motivation to do it on your own, which many people don't, I highly recommend the buddy system.

You have a body that is physically more appealing than most 20 years olds. If you could give one piece of advice to help others reach their dream bodies, what would it be?

Besides the obvious (diet), hit the weights. Muscle burns fat; it doesn't get much simpler than that. For me, the missing piece for years was lack of weight training in my workout regime. When I finally incorporated weight training, my body leaned out very quickly. Simply put, the more muscle your body has, the higher your metabolism. So, go heavy or go home!

How often do you workout, and what is a typical workout?

I workout 4 to 5 times a week, and it's always great if I can get a bonus sixth day in.

Sample workout:

10 min. of treadmill warm up
  2 min. fast paced walk at incline of 2
  2 min. at incline of 10
  2 min. walking backwards at incline of 10
  3 min. jogging at incline of 2
  1 min. of fast paced walk at incline of 2

Follow this warm up with a few minutes of dynamic warmup targeting the muscles I will use in my workout.

30 to 45 minutes of weight training

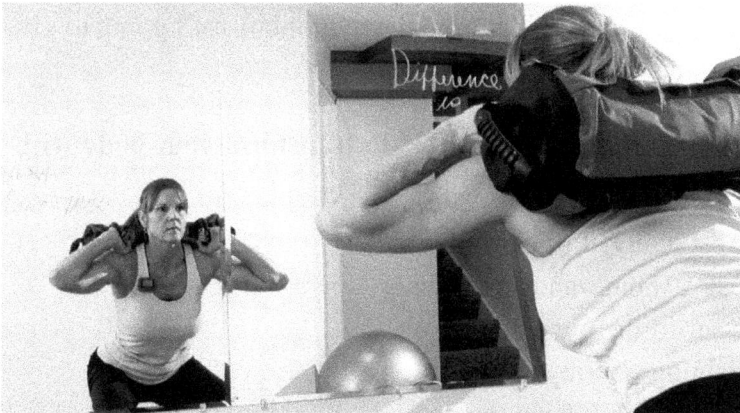

Bonus/optional:10 to 20 minutes of HIIT:
  Tabata style 50 sec. work/10 sec. rest
    - sandbag burpees
    - lateral hop over sandbag with a tuck jump
    - push up with a sandbag drag

- Sandbag squats or squat jumps
- traveling alternating lunges with sandbag overhead
- jump rope

Cool down

Also, I love my pink sandbag; it is one of my favorite pieces of workout equipment, along with my adjustable dumbbells and interval timer. If I were stranded on a deserted island, I would want those those items.

No matter what type of workout you are doing, always push past your comfort zone. It is the point at which you really want to quit and you feel like you can't do another rep that the exercise is most effective and things really start working.

It is all about intensity, asking your body to do things it hasn't done before and then responding by pushing past your comfort zone and leaving it all at the gym (or in the basement in my case). Just going through the motions isn't going to give you the result you're looking for.

Do you think it is possible to transform your body without going to the gym?

Absolutely! I prefer to workout at home and really only went to the gym when I was training for my competition since I didn't have the necessary leg equipment to achieve the look I wanted. It is much more convenient for me, and I workout at a much greater intensity, when I am at home.

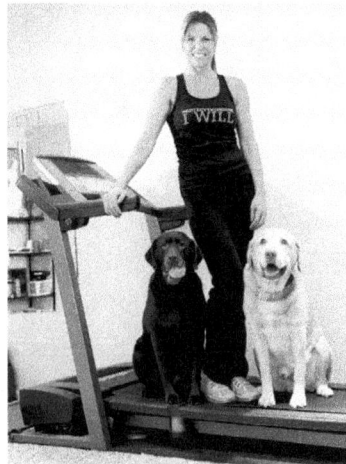

At the gym, I find it difficult when I have to wait for a piece of equipment or have to alter my workout. At home, the only ones who get in my way are my dogs, Graham and Gracie, who like to drop balls on the treadmill when I'm running and try to lay on my mat when I'm doing abs.

I do enjoy group fitness classes but obviously can't get that in my home gym. My version of group fitness classes are workout videos. I spend a lot of time watching previews of videos online and reading reviews before I purchase them. I research what programs are best suited for me and my goals and will also keep me motivated. While the actual workout is important, for me, the other two critical components are the instructor and the music.

I will have to give a shout out here to one of my favorite motivators and fitness inspirations: Chalene Johnson. While I enjoy her "Turbo Jam" and "Turbo Fire" cardio kickboxing videos, it was "Chalean Extreme" that got me hooked on weight training. This series changed my philosophy that weight training was boring.

I always knew the importance of weight training, but when I saw my body leaning out after just 30 days, it finally hit home. If you're worried that it is too expensive to purchase a lot of weight equipment, no need to worry. One of my best fitness purchases, and most frequently used pieces of equipment, is a set of adjustable dumbbells (I use PowerBlock dumbbells that go from 3 to 24 lbs each), which I purchased for roughly $180.

For many reasons, going to the gym just wasn't the best fit for me. In order to remain committed to my health and fitness, I had to find something that worked for me. At first, it was difficult to workout at home because of the many distractions (kids, spouse, phone calls, dinner, laundry). I learned to schedule my workout time or "me time." "Me time" meant if I was down in my workout room, no one could bother me. If it wasn't life threatening, it could wait till I was done working out; and "I'm hungry" is not life threatening.

Now that my workouts are scheduled at 4:30 a.m., there are no interruptions.

How have your workouts changed compared to your 20s or 30s?

Workouts from my 20s until recently were almost entirely cardio based. My workout philosophy was cardio, cardio, and more cardio. In addition to getting into aerobics in my college years, I also became an avid biker and runner.

Anyone who is a runner knows how addicting it is. My workouts were either entirely running or had running incorporated into them (for example, cardio kickboxing followed by a run). I attempted, on a number of occasions, to incorporate a weight-training program but never stuck to it. I felt if I wasn't running or jumping around working up a sweat, I wasn't getting a good workout.

Now, my workout schedule now is more like 80% weight training and 20% cardio, which is a drastic change. I

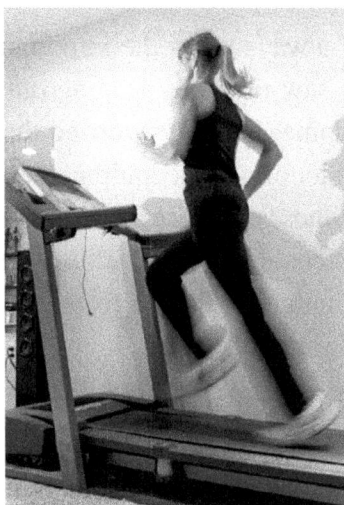

was what I have heard Rob say a number of times: a skinny fat person. Now I'm older, wiser, and much leaner. Who says you can't teach an old dog a new trick?

If you could give one piece of advice about your nutrition plan, what would it be?

Journaling is the number one tool for a successful diet.

I was not familiar with eating fruits or vegetables, and I still struggle today with getting them into my diet. While working out comes so easy to me, it is this area that I find difficult.

One of the most important things I have learned is that you need to make sure you are eating every 3 to 4 hours, whether it is a meal or a snack, and try to incorporate carbs, proteins and fats into every meal. It may take some time to figure out the perfect ratio for your body, but it is time well spent.

While many people use ratios such as 40% carbs, 40% protein and 20% fat, it is also recommended to figure at least 1g of protein per pound body weight, .35g fat per pound body weight, and the rest carbs. I know you just wanted one piece of advice, but I also know that without journaling my food, my nutrition plan would not have succeeded.

Many women have struggled with a weight problem their whole lives, which is sometimes psychological. Have you ever struggled with a weight problem or were you one of those people who could eat whatever you wanted and not gain a pound?

While in reality I never had a weight problem, psychologically, I had a weight problem.

As a child and all through high school, I was a junk-food junkie. I ate whatever I wanted when I wanted. I remember going to McDonalds, and my typical order was a Big Mac (sometimes two), a large strawberry shake, and a cinnamon roll. I could easily polish off a whole box of cereal in one sitting, especially Peanut Butter Cap'n Crunch, and my Dad and I had ice cream for a snack almost every night. My parents tried desperately to get me to eat fruit and vegetables, but I just wouldn't (thank goodness my dog liked them). Weight was never a problem for me—until I left for college, that is.

About a week before everyone was leaving for college, I was at a party when a male friend of mine said. "I guess when I see you next, you will be 15 lbs. heavier." I was very confused and said "Why?" He said, "Haven't you heard of the 'freshman 15'? When girls go to college, they gain at least 15 lbs." If learning that I was going to gain 15 pounds wasn't enough, I also learned that my Dad was diagnosed with colon cancer. I was starting the exciting next stage of my life scared I was going to gain weight and lose my father.

For the first time in my young life, the future seemed very scary, and things were spinning out of control. Food, or lack thereof, became a way for me to try and control my life. I developed severe eating disorders that were a part of my life for the next six years. I initially was anorexic, but, over the course of the next few years, as people tried to control my anorexia, I developed bulimia. While everyone told me how sick I looked, I thought I looked great. I worked out several times a day and, over the course of the day, would eat one Little Debbie Nutty Bar, saving the second bar in the pack for the next day.

Needless to say, my parents weren't very happy that I wasted thousands of dollars on the university meal plan. My first summer home from college, I weighed 99 pounds. Since I was now home, my parents saw what was going on, and they started to intervene and force me to eat. This was traumatic, and I needed a plan or I was going to gain weight. I started to record every calories I consumed and would workout enough to burn more than I ate.

My dad eventually took my bike away and monitored my exercise and my eating. Because I was now being forced to eat and my exercise was being monitored, I needed a new plan, and bulimia seemed liked a good one at the time. I was going to be the one in control.

By the time I went back to college that fall, I had everyone fooled. This horrible disease continued to progress for the next three years. I loved my position as an aerobics instructor at the university but was asked to step down because I had gotten so thin and was not portraying a healthy image. My manager at the time knew exactly what was going on and finally contacted my roommates and my parents.

Bulimia had taken over my life, and I finally agreed to seek help. I left school and was admitted to a treatment facility in Milwaukee, where I stayed for a month while I gained 30 pounds to reach what they considered to be my goal weight.

In reality, I was not overweight, but in my head I was. I did not like what I saw in the mirror. My recovery was an on-again/off-again struggle, and I completely fell off the wagon after my father passed away in 1989. It wasn't until the day in 1991 when I found out I was pregnant that I seemed to be instantly cured.

How quickly things change when you have another life to think about. I continued to workout throughout my pregnancy but was very anxious about how I would react after the baby was born and had all that baby weight to deal with. Thankfully, the weight came off very quickly with exercise, and I did not resort back to the bulimic or anorexic ways.

My next two pregnancies went the same, and I was very fortunate to get my pre-pregnancy body back fairly quickly. It was not until 13 years later that I once again struggled with bulimia. The stress of life, kids, work, finances, unfulfilling relationship, et cetera, had me down. I used bulimia as a way to gain back control. Thankfully, this episode was very short lived, and, with a little life coaching, I was able to get things back on track and have never gone back.

How do you know how many calories you should eat each day? Do you count them?

I typically do not count calories but focus on my percentages of proteins, carbs and fats in each meal. In 2012, I took a MetaCheck, metabolic rate test, to measure precisely how many calories my body was burning and determine how many calories I should eat to lose or maintain weight. According to my test, I could eat 2,193 calories to maintain my weight with only 30 minutes of moderate exercise a day.

During my competition training, I had to be pretty strict with my eating plan so had to monitor my calories as well as carbs, proteins and fats. I started my training at about 1,500 calories a day. After 2 weeks at 1,500, I was leaning out too quickly and had to up my calories. With the heavy weight training, my body became a fat-burning machine, and I was eventually eating about 2,200 calories a day. But not 2,200 calories of whatever I wanted: I was eating a lean, clean diet.

I figured out a 1,500-calorie eating plan and a 2,200-calorie eating plan and would monitor where my body was at and where I needed to be calorie-wise. I do not count calories now but have a good idea where I'm at without actually counting them.

I would definitely recommend the metabolic test in order to find out how many calories your body is burning. Then, you can lay out your plan depending whether you want to lose, gain or maintain weight. One thing I can't stress enough: Journal everything you're eating. After a couple weeks of journaling, you should have a pretty good idea of what modifications you need to make based on the changes your body has or has not made. Soon your healthy-eating plan becomes habit, a way of life, and you will know basically where you're at without actually counting out each calorie.

What is your favorite healthy recipe?

My favorite healthy recipe is my breakfast omelet/wrap

5 egg whites
3 cherry tomatoes
1/3 c. (or a couple slices) of avocado
½ - 1 c. baby spinach
Mrs. Dashes seasonings

Mix all the above in nutri bullet and pour on a hot griddle, cooking for about 5 minutes on each side.

Top with salsa (and shredded cheese when not in competition mode) and eat like an omelet or make it a wrap (I use Joseph's Flax Oat Bran and Whole Wheat Lavash Bread)

What motivates you to keep going?

The feeling I get from working out is a huge motivator. It's more than the physical benefits of improving my cardiovascular health, building muscle, and keeping my body looking good. I feel totally renewed after a workout and sometime can't even remember what I might have been worried or stressed out about when I started the workout.

Working out relieves my stress and anxiety, improves my mood, gives me energy and helps me sleep better, just to name a few benefits. On days when I need a little push to get going, I think about how great I feel after a workout.

I also use motivational quotes to keep me going. I recently bought chalk markers and I use them to write motivational statements on my workout mirrors and bathroom mirrors.

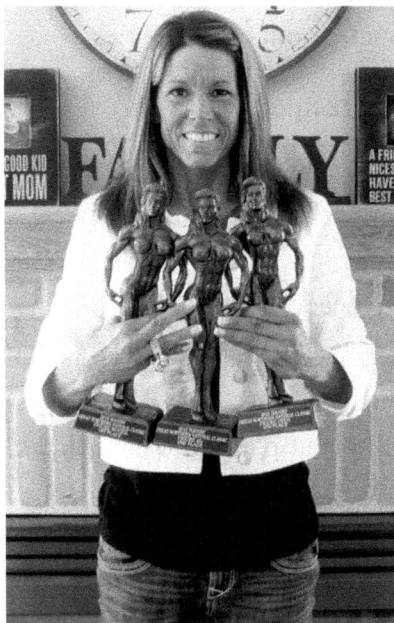

Sometimes when I am struggling to push out my last few reps, I will look up at my mirror to see the words "One More," and it will motivate me to dig a little deeper. More often than not, I will even get more than just one more rep out.

Setting your goals and expending the effort has its rewards.

How would you respond to any one of the common excuses women use not to workout?

No matter which one excuse I hear, it is just that, an excuse. An excuse serves the simple purpose of relieving us from the guilt associated with not doing what we said we were going to do. If you really want something, you will make it happen instead of making excuses.

You always hear sayings such as "How badly do you want it?" I don't think it is how badly you want it, I think it is how hard you are willing to work to get it.

You need to do yourself a favor and make time to exercise and not make excuses. Remember this quote, "Those who do not make time to exercise will need to make time for illness."

What advice would you give to women in their 40s?

The important thing is to know exactly what you want to achieve. Whether you are 20 or 60, it doesn't matter. Age is a number, not an excuse. Do you want to run a marathon? Do you want to look great in your bikini on the beach in Mexico? Do you want to compete in a figure competition?

Whatever it is that you want to achieve, make a plan, and go for it. Goals do not have age limits. I like to use the SCAMPI approach for setting goals. SCAMPI is an acronym that will increase your chances of success.

S - Specific – Set specific goals that are clearly defined. For example, not just I want to lose weight, but I want to lose 15 pounds by a certain date, and I will do it by improving my diet and working out 4 days a week.

C - Challenging – Set goals that are challenging. Make sure your goals are not too easily accomplished but realistic and challenging enough.

A - Approach – Set your goal with a positive mindset. Instead of saying that you want to lose weight because you don't want to be fat, say you want to lose weight because you will look and feel better.

M - Measurable – Find a way to assess the progress you are making. Saying I want to look better is not attainable. Saying I want to lose 3% body fat in 4 weeks is measurable.

P - Proximal – Break down your bigger goal into smaller goals. If you want to lose 20 pounds in the next 6 months, break it down into how much you need to lose each week or each month.

I - Inspirational – Keep your goal in line with your own ideas and inspirations. Be sure to set the goal for you and no one else.

My typical 1500 calorie day:

Breakfast:	Breakfast wrap
	5 egg whites
	1/3 c. avocado
	1 c. spinach
	3 cherry tomatoes
	1 Joseph's whole wheat lavash wrap
Snack:	Quest Protein Bar
Lunch:	½ c. brown rice
	4 oz. chicken breast

Snack:	Plain rice cake (unsalted) with
	1 TBSP almond butter and an apple
Dinner:	8 oz cod with Mrs. Dash Seasoning
	1 med. Sweet potato with cinnamon
Snack:	Chocolate Peanut Butter
	Protein drink or Quest Bar

Supplements:	Advocare – OmegaPlex
	Advocare – Coreplex Multi Vitamin
	Advocare – Argenine Extreme

Typical Competition Workout Schedule:

Day 1: Back and Abs
Day 2: Hamstrings and Glutes
Day 3: Shoulders
Day 4: Arms and Abs
Day 5: Quads and Calves
Day 6: Chest and Abs

½ hour of cardio each day rotating between HIIT, Stair Climber, treadmill interval sprinting

And that's how they did it!

Eating plans used by Mary and Cheryl

We started Mary out in Phase I. Here original calorie needs were 1667 calories, so we put her into a small caloric deficit of 10% below her maintenance intake of 1667, which was 1500 calories per day. This plan worked well for the majority of her transformation. As she started getting lean, we had to re-evaluate her daily energy needs. I highly recommend updating your calorie needs as you transform your body because as you add muscle and lose fat, your metabolism changes. What you used for your calorie count on day one will probably be a bit different as you approach your goal.

Clean 1500 calories Phase 1

Breakfast		Protein	Carbs	Fat	Calories
4	egg white	14.39	0.96	0.22	63.36
1 Cup	Oat meal	13.2	55.8	6	297
1/2 C	tomato	0.76	4.18	0.3	19
	TOTALS	28.35	60.94	6.52	379.36
Lunch					
1/3 C	Black beans	3.81	10.2	0.23	56.76
1 Cup	Brown Rice-Cooked	4.9	49.7	1.2	232
3 oz	Chicken Breast	19.5	0	1.2	93
1 Cup	Vegetables-Mixed	5.2	23.8	0.2	108
	TOTALS	33.41	83.7	2.83	489.76
Snack					
1 Cup	Allmond Milk	1	2	3.5	40
1 Cup	Blueberries	0.54	10.51	0.25	41.33
1 Scoop	Isopure Protein	25	0	0.5	105
	TOTALS	26.54	12.51	4.24	186.33
Dinner					
3 oz	Salmon-Broiled	18.81	0	10.5	174
2 Cup	Asparagus	9.2	15.2	1.2	88
1TBL	Olive oil	0	0	14	130
	TOTALS	28.01	15.2	25.7	392
TOTALS for the day		116.31	172.35	39.29	1447.45
		35%	50%	25%	

130

Below was Cheryl's first eating program for her competition, approximately 1500 calories, had a good resemblance to Phase 2. We eventually had to boost her up to over 2,000 calories and cut out her cardiovascular training because she started to get too lean due to putting on more muscle. Eating more, working out less, and still getting lean is a problem any women would love to have. She earned this by adding the intense weight training to her program.

Breakfast		Protein	Carbs	Fats	Calories
1 C	avocados	0.88	3.74	6.42	70.08
5	egg whites	17.5	1.5		85
64g	Josephs whole wheat wrap	10	14	4	100
1 C	Spinach, raw	0.86	1.09	0.12	6.9
34 g	cherry tomatoes	0.27	1.02	0.14	6.12
	TOTALS	29.51	21.35	10.68	268.1
Snack					
1	Quest chocolate brownine bar	20	24	6	170
	TOTALS	20	24	6	170
Lunch					
1/2 C	Brown Rice, cooked	2.45	24.85	0.6	116
4 oz	Chicken Breast	26	0	1.6	124
	TOTALS	28.45	24.85	2.2	240
Snack					
2	Celery stalks	1	4	0	20
1 TBL	Almond Butter	2.41	3.4	9.46	101.28
	TOTALS	3.41	7.4	9.46	121.28
Dinner					
8 oz	Fish-Cod	54	0	2	240
1	Sweet potato- medium	2.29	23.61	0.17	102.6
	TOTALS	56.29	23.61	2.17	342.6
Snack					
1 scoop	Whey protein	21	1	0	90
1	Quest Peanut butter supreme	20	21	10	210
28.5 g	Creatine	0	21.5		100
	TOTALS	41	4305	10	400
	Daily TOTALS	178.66	144.71	40.51	1542
		45%	35%	25%	

The phase 3 plan is what Mary used at the end of her program. She still had a few stubborn pounds of fat to lose. So days 1-3 she ate a 1200 calorie lower carb plan (20% defecit) to really try to tap into and melt away stored body fat. Then to keep her body from going haywire, she introduced carbs back in on day four and did a 20% surplus in her calorie count. This kept her body from thinking it was starving and continued to get results. The final 2 weeks of her program she just used the low carb eating plan (the deficit) This type of eating is not typically done for more than a few weeks.

Phase 3, the deficit Example of day 1,2, and 3						
Breakfast			Protein	Carbs	Fat	
6	Each	Egg Whites	21	1.8	0	102
1	Cup	Spinach	0.86	1.09	0.12	6.9
	TOTALS	Grams	21.86	2.89	0.12	108.9
Snack						
1	Scoop	Protein Powder	23	3	2	120
0.3	TBL	Peanut Butter	1.2	0.9	2.4	31.5
	TOTALS		24.2	3.9	4.4	151.5
Lunch						
1	Cup	Cabbage. Red. Raw	1.27	6.56	0.14	27.59
1	Cup	Cucumber, slices	0.8	2.8	0	14
0.5	Cup	Lettuce	0.25	0.82	0.04	3.85
1	Each	Morning star grillers, vegan	12	7	2.5	100
1	2' dia 5'long	Sweet Potato, cooked	2.29	23.61	0.17	104.88
½	Cup	Diced tomatoes	0.76	4.18	0.3	19
	TOTALS		17.37	44.97	3.15	269.32
Snack						
1	Each	Trader Joes reduced carb tortilla	4	10	0	45
5	Ounces	Tuna in water	25	0	1.67	150
	TOTALS		29	10	150	195
Dinner						
1	Cup	Broccoli	5.7	9.84	0.22	51.52
6	ounces	Fish, Baked Cod	38.8	0	1.4	178
1	TBL	Oil, Gapesced	0	0	13.6	120.22
	TOTALS		44.5	9.84	15.22	349.74
Snack						
1	TBL	Peanut Butter	4	3	8	105
1	Scoop	Protein Powder	15	4	1	70
	TOTALS		155.93	78.6	33.56	1249.46
			~45%	~25%	~25%	

Phase 3, the surplus, Example of day 4						
Breakfast						
1	Cup	Oatmeal-measured uncooked	13.2	55.8	6	297
1	Scoop	Protein Powder	15	4	1	70
		TOTALS				
Snack						
4	Ounces	Black Beans	9	26.88	0.6	152
1	Cup	Lettuce	0.49	1.63	0.08	7.7
1/2	Cup	Tomato-Diced	0.76	4.18	0.3	19
1	Each	Trader Joes low carb Tortilla	4	10	0	45
0.3	Cup	Cheddar Cheese-Shredded	7.03	0.36	9.36	113.85
		TOTALS				
Lunch						
2	Ounces	Barilla Pasta	7	42	1	200
1	Cup	Brocolli	5.7	9.84	0.22	51.52
4	Ounces	Fish-Baked Tilapia	21	0	1	93
		TOTALS	33.7	51.84	2.22	344.52
Snack						
0.5	Cup	Oatmeal-measured uncooked	6.6	27.9	3	148.5
1	Scoop	Protein Powder	15	4	1	70
		TOTALS	21.6	31.9	4	218.5
Dinner						
1	Cup	Beans-Green	2.2	7.75	0.46	44.4
4	Ounces	Fish-Baked Cod	25.87	0	0.93	118.67
1	Medium	Sweet Potato	2.07	26.76	0.21	114.76
		TOTALS	44.5	9.84	15.22	349.74
Snack						
2	TBL	Peanut Butter	8	6	16	210
1	Scoops	Protein Powder	25	5	5	122.5
		TOTALS	147	230	38	1777
			~30%	~50%	~20%	

Need more help with choosing foods that will fit into your daily eating plan?

There are many Apps or online programs that will track everything you eat. You can set up your macronutrient percentages for the day.(i.e. carbohydrates 40%, protein 40%, fat 20%) They will even track your calories, vitamins, and minerals. The neatest thing is that some of these programs will even allow you to scan in the barcode of the foods that you have eaten. Just make sure to watch your serving sizes. Best of all, they are free programs.

NOTE: Don't worry too much about making each meal the perfect percentages of macronutrients, just try to get close for the entire day.

Here are some of my favorite helpful Apps/programs/websites:

My Fitness Pal (great free App for tracking food intake)

SparkPeople.com (nice community of people with lots of support)

RealHealthyRecipies.com (free downloadable recipe book)

Strength Workouts
Periodization Table for Resistance Training

2-4 Reps 3-5 sets	5-6 Reps 3-5 sets	8-12 Reps 3-5 sets	15 + Reps 3-5 sets
Power	Strength	Hypertrophy (building)	Endurance

Rest 3-5 minutes	Rest 2-3 minutes	Rest 60-90 seconds	Rest 30-45 seconds
		Best place to be for transformation	

Getting results with strength training is really very simple. Choose your goal; power, strength, hypertrophy, or endurance and workout each body part to the guidelines above.

The **hypertrophy** stage is best used to build quality muscle for women or anyone for that matter. The power phase is used more with athletes to get them explosive. Not saying it couldn't help with a women trying to transform their body. It's just not the most efficient way of putting on muscle to increase metabolism for beginners. In extreme cases like with Mary, we chose to use the hypertrophy phase for her upper body and endurance phase for her lower body because we didn't want to build more muscle in her legs. Her legs grew quickly in the hypertrophy phase and made her physique look awkward. The key is to continually change from one stage to the next so you don't get hurt or peak. An example would be to work out in the hypertrophy stage for 8 weeks, then the endurance stage for 2 weeks, and finally take a break and cross train for a week while enjoying swimming, hiking or any other exercise you enjoy. Then start all over again. Periodization can be a chapter all by itself. The point is that if you stay in the hypertrophy stage and continually add more weight to your workout, you will eventually get hurt.

Sample Beginner Workout-3 days per week, Nonconsecutive days

At Home	In the Gym
The simple seven	**The simple seven**
1. Squat with Dumbbells	1. Leg Press Machine
2. Row with bands or Dumbbells	2. Lat Pulldown Machine
3. Chest press with band or DB	3. Chest Press Machine or DB
4. Shoulder press with DB	4. Shoulder Press Machine or DB
5. Bicep curl with band or Db	5. Biceps curl with barbell
6. Tricep extension with band or DB	6. Tricep pushdown on pulley
7. Ab crunch	7. Ab crunch on physioball

When not competing, Cheryl likes to do workout videos at **www.cathe.com** "I get cathe on demand and cathe live (which is a live class each week) for $19.97 a month. Her workouts are phenomenal. She also provides on her main website a tab called rotations and she makes monthly rotations (workouts suggests for 6 days a week for 4 weeks)." Mary likes to use the free website bodyrock.tv for more variety in her workouts.

The free Nike fit app is a good addition to add variety to your workouts.

DailyBurn.com offers a free 30 day trial to their on demand workouts.

Workouts

Mary's sample strength workouts (medium intensity)

This workout alternated upper body and lower body three times throughout the week.

	Monday	Tuesday	Wednesday	Thursday	Friday	Saturday	Sunday
Week 1	Upper		Lower		Upper		
Week 2	Lower		Upper		Lower		

Upper Body A

EXERCISE:	Set 1	Set 2	Set 3	Set 4	Set 5	Set 6
Walking Pushups	max reps	max reps	max reps			
Pike Push ups	max reps	max reps	max reps			
Dips on the floor	max reps	max reps	max reps			
Write down your total	reps	No Rest	between set	, 6 min cycle!		
Shoulder Press	5lb x 15	5lb x 12	5lb x 10			
Lateral Raise	5lb x 15	5lb x 12	5lb x 10			
Lat Pull Down	x12	x10	x8			
Seated Cable Row	x12	x10	x8			
Straight arm Pull down						
DB bicep curl	x12	x10	x8			
Db overhead tricep ext	x12	x10	x8			
Reverse Crunch	20 sec.	20 sec.	20 sec.			
Bicycle Crunch	20 sec.	20 sec.	20 sec.			
Plank Hold	Failure	Failure	Failure			

Lower Body A

EXERCISE:	Set 1	Set 2	Set 3	Set 4	Set 5	Set 6
Frog Hops	x15	x15	15			
Walking Deadlifts	5lb x15	5lb x15	5lb x15			
Body wt. Squats	15	15	15			
6 min. cycle through	all	3 exercises	as many	times as possible		
Physio ball leg curl	x15	x15	x15			
PB Hip Lifts	x15	x15	x15			
Pb St. leg Glute lift	x15	x15	x15			
Med Ball Leg Extension	x20	x20	x20			
Med ball Leg Curl	x20	x20	x20			
Super Man	20 sec.	20 sec.	20 sec.			
Bent Knee Crunch	20 sec.	20 sec.	20 sec.			
Plank Hold	Failure	Failure	Failure			

137

In this workout Mary went from 3 days of strength training to a four day per week split. She worked synergistic muscle groups (muscles that work together) two days per week.

Monday	Tuesday	Wednesday	Thursday	Friday	Saturday	Sunday
Workout 1	Workout 2		Workout 1	Workout 2		

4 day split routine

Workout 1 Chest/Shoulders/Triceps

EXERCISE:	Set 1	Set 2	Set 3	Set 4	Set 5	Set 6
CHEST:						
Band Assisted Pushups	Failure	Failure	Failure			
DB Incline Chest Press	12lbs x 12	15lbs x 10	17.5lbs x 8			
Shoulders:						
DB Arnold Presses	10lb x 15	10lb x 12	12lb x 10			
Windmills	5lb x 15	5lb x 15	5lb x 15			
Cable lateral Raise	20lb x 15	20lb x 12	20lb x 10			
Triceps:						
Dips off bench	Failure	Failure	Failure			
Rope extesnions(rope)	30lbs x 15	30lbs x 12	30lbs x 10			
1 arm cable underhand ext	20lbs x 15	20lbs x12	20 lbs x 10			
extension(each arm)						
Leg Drops (abs)	45 sec.	30 sec.	30 sec			
Windshield washers	x15/side	x15/side	x15/side			

Workout 2 Back/Biceps/Legs

EXERCISE:	Set 1	Set 2	Set 3	Set 4	Set 5	Set 6
Back:						
T-Bar Row						
Assisted PU w/band						
Biceps:						
Barbell Curl 2/0/4 tempo	20lbs x 15	20lbs x12	20 lbs x 10			
Legs:						
Body Weight Squats	x 50	x 60	x 70			
Plie DB Squats	15lbs x 25	15lbs x 20	15lbs x 15			
1 leg Bridges	x15	x15	x12			
Jackknife	x20	x20	x20			
Physio Ball Crunch	Failure	Failure	Failure			
Plank Hold	Failure	Failure	Failure			

Sample of Cheryl's 6 day workout plan (high intensity)

Monday	Tuesday	Wednesday	Thursday	Friday	Saturday	Sunday
Back/Abs	Hams/Glutes	Shoulders	Arms/abs	Quads/calves	Chest/abs	

This workout is a bit more time consuming and demanding. It requires working out 6 days per week and hitting each muscle group once per week but very intensely. It's not that it's too difficult for anyone to do, just takes a little bit more dedication in your already busy schedule. As you recall from Cheryl's story, she typically did this at a 4 a.m. so there were no excuses.

Day 1 - Back and Abs

EXERCISE:	Set 1	Set 2	Set 3	Set 4	Set 5	Set 6	Set 7
Pull Ups (to failure)							
Bent Over BB Row	x 25	add # x 15-20	add # x 10-12	x 10-12	x 10-12	x 10-12	
Rev. Grip							
Seated Cable Row	x 25	add # x 15-20	add # x 8-10	x 8-10	x 8-10		
Plank Row R	x15	x15	x15				
Plank Row L	x15	x15	x15				
Hyperextension	x 15-20	x 15-20	x 15-20				
*use lower back not							
glutes!!							
Bicycles	x 30-40	x30-40	x30-40	x30-40	x30-40		
Straight Leg Crunch	x 20-25	x20-25	x20-25	x20-25	x 20-25		
*** no rest inbetween bicycles and crunches - rest 20-30 seconds after sl crunch only before							
starting next set.							

Day 2 Hames & Glutes

	Set 1	Set 2	Set 3	Set 4	Set 5	Set 6
SLDL (keep lbs. same)	x8-12	x8-12	x8-12	x8-12		
* start with 50#	50# x 12	60# x 12	60# x 12	50# x 12		
Lying Leg Curls	x15	x15	x15			
40# good weights	30# x 15	35# x 12	40# x 15			
Walking Lunges or Bulgarian	x15	x15	x15			
15# weights	x 15 each	x 15 each	bulg. x 15			
Single Leg Bridge R	x 15-20	x 15-20	x 15-20			
with 12.5 # weight	x20	x20	x20			
Single Leg Bridge L	x 15-20	x 15-20	x 15-20			
	x20	x20	x20			
Cable Kick Backs R	x 12-18	x 12-18	x 12-18	x 12-18		
	10# x 18	12.5 # x 12	12.5 x 18	12.5 x 20		
Cable Kick Backs L	x 12-18	x 12-18	x 12-18	x 12-18		
Back to back no rest	10# x 18	12.5 # x 12	12.5 x 18	12.5 x 20		
Seated/Standing Calf Raises	x 25	x25	x23			
Free Motion Machine	40# x 25	50# x 25	60# x 25			

Notes: Warm up on a Treadmill 10 minutes / Stair Climber 20 minutes
***last set of kickbacks did standing leg curl 12.5 x 20

139

Day 3 - Shoulders
March 6, 2013

EXERCISE:	Set 1	Set 2	Set 3	Set 4	Set 5	Set 6
One Arm DB Press	1x20	1x20	1x20			
L	1x20	1x20	1x20			
*Keep switching from R to L no rest at all until complete with all 3 sets!						
Side DB Laterals	x15-25	x15-25	x15-25	x15-25	x15-25	x15-25
*Keep weight the same on all 6 sets						
Seated Bent Over DB	x20-25	x20-25	x20-25	x20-25	x20-25	
Raise (rear delt.)						
*Keep weight the same on all 5 sets						
Seated DB Press	x10	x10	x10	x10		
Seated Alt. DB Press	x20	x20	x20	x20		
*Do 10 DB Press both arms then 20 alt with no rest in between-rest 30-60 sec. after alternating						
Walkie Planks	20 sec.	20 sec.	20 sec.			
Plank Hold	Failure	Failure	Failure			
Hold to failure						
*Perform Walkie Planks then directly to plank hold-no rest until failure then rest 30-60 sec.						
Patty Cake Planks	20 sec.	20 sec.	20 sec.			
Plank Hold	Failure	Failure	Failure			
Hold to failure						
*Perform Patty Cake Planks then directly to plank hold-no rest until failure then rest 30-60 sec.						
Notes:						

My own notes:
Start off with 10-12 on presses
Laterals and Deltoids go down in weight

Day 4 Arms - Abs   only about 30-45 sec. rest
March 21, 2013

EXERCISE:	Set 1	Set 2	Set 3	Set 4	Set 5
Barbell Curl	x 8-12	x 8-12	x8-12	x 8-12	
weights plus bar 3/21	25# x 12	26# x 10	26# x 8	26# x 8	
Hammer Curls	x 8-12	x 8-12	x8-12	x 8-12	
	12# x 12	15# x 10	15# x 9	15# x 10	
Alternating DB Curls	x 8-12	x 8-12	x8-12	x 8-12	
Incline****	12 x 20	12 x 20	12 x 20	15# x 10	
Cable Skull Crushers	x 8-12	x 8-12	x8-12	x 8-12	x 8-12
*lying on bench 3/21	10# x 15	15# x 12	15# x 12	18# x 10	
Cable Press Downs	x 8-12	x 8-12	x8-12	x 8-12	x 8-12
Bar 3/21/13	18# x 12	21# x 12	25# x 12	25# x 8	25# x 9
Rope Kick Outs	x12-15	x12-15	x12-15		
go a little lighter	15# x 12	15# x 12	15# x 12		
Ab Circuit					
Rev Crunch	x20	x20	x20	x20	
Flutter Kicks	x50	x50	x50	x50	
Bicycles	x20	x20	x20	x20	
Crunches	x30	x30	x30	x30	
* no rest until after crunches then rest only 30-60 seconds and repeat for 4 sets total					

140

Day 5 Quads & Calves

EXERCISE:	Set 1	Set 2	Set 3	Set 4	Set 5	Set 6
Wide Squat	x10	x10	x10	x10	x10	x10
keep same weight	55#	65# x 10	65# x 10	65# x 10	65# x 10	65# x 10
Side Squat (alt r/l)	x30	x30	x30			
keep same weight	15# x 30	15# x 30	15# x 30			
Hack Squats	x25	+ x 20	+ x 15	+ x 10	- x 30	
close stance	50# x 25	60# x 20	70# x 15	90# x 15	#60 x 30	
Walking Lunges	x30	x30	x30			
w/ dumbells 30#	30# x 30	30# x 30	30# x 30			
go immediately to	30 sec	30 sec	30 sec			
Toe Taps						
Leg Extension	x 20-25	x 20-25	x 20-25			
toes in then directly	20# x 15	20# x 20	20# x 22			
to squat jumps	30 s.j.	30 s.j.	30 s.j.			
Seated Calf Raise	x 30	x 20	x 10 + burn	x 10 + burn		
*add 10 burns to 2 sets	25# x 30	25# x 25	25# x 10	25# x 10		
Standing Calf Raise	x 25	x25	x25			
+10 burns on each	40# x 25	#50 x 25 +	50# x 25 +			

Day 6 Chest and Abs

EXERCISE:	Set 1	Set 2	Set 3	Set 4	Set 5	Set 6
Hi Incline Chest Press	x30	x18-20	x12-15	x10-12	x 6-8	x 6-8
Dumbbells	6# x 30	8# x 20	9# x 20	#12 x 15	15# x 12	#15 x 15
Need to start heavier next time						
Bench Push Ups	30 sec.	30 sec.	30 sec.			
immediately to						
Patty Cakes	30 sec.	30 sec.	30 sec.			
ABS:						
Hanging Knee Raises	x15	x15	x15	x15		
Russian Twist	x30	x30	x30	x30		
Cable Crunch	x20	x20	x20	x20		
Vacuum	x 5	x 5	x 5	x 5		
Only rest between sets						
* I did a 10 min. Chalean Abs also						

Notes:
Cardio: 20 + min. on treadmill and Elliptical

141

Cardiovascular training for your body transformation

Before starting any workout program you should make sure to have a medical clearance from your doctor. The latest cardiovascular training advice offered by the American Heart Association is to get 30 minutes of moderate-intensity aerobic training 5 days per week for a total of 150 minutes or 25 minutes of vigorous activity three days per week for a total of 75 minutes. Intensity is the key to your cardio workouts when trying to transform your body.

The most effective form of cardio for burning fat is HIIT (high intensity interval training). If you step on a piece of cardio equipment and you feel like you didn't even break a sweat you're probably not doing your cardio hard enough.

Although there is no specific formula to HIIT, a common strategy involves a 2:1 ratio of work to recovery, for example 30 seconds of hard sprinting alternated with 15 seconds of walking or jogging. The entire HIIT session may last between ten and thirty minutes.

Example:

Level	Time in minutes	Target heart rate %
Beginner	2	65%
	1	85%
	2	65%
	1	85%
	2	65%
	1	85%
	2	65%
	1	85%

As with any part of your workout, you need to keep your cardio plans changing. Your body adapts very quickly. So mix it up. For a more intense workout, try HIIT. If you are just beginning try a steady walk for 30-40 minutes in your training zone. You could also exercise to a work-out video or take a class at your gym. Instead of the treadmill try the bike. For something different head down to the school track and do some sprints. For overall fat loss try to get at least 3-5 cardiovascular work-outs per week. Remember, you can't out train your diet. You can only get leaner by decreasing calories and/or increasing activity. DON'T become a cardio addict!

HIIT	General Cardio@ 60-85% of target zone
3-5 days per week	3-5 days per week
10-30 minutes/day	30-40 minutes/day

Here's how the American Council on Exercise (ACE) views body fat percentage norms.

It's important to note that the scale weight in and of itself doesn't always paint the best picture for your success. After time goes on and you start to put on some quality muscle, which isn't a bad thing, you may gain muscle mass and lose fat and the scale may not move. Remember the picture of the fat vs muscle? Muscle is much denser and takes up much less space than the same volume of fat. So have a trained professional take your body fat measurements when you start losing a lot of weight so you don't get discouraged about your progress.

ACE Body Fat % Norms		
Description	Women	Men
Essential Fat	10-13%	2-5%
Athletes	14-20%	6-13%
Fitness	21-24%	14-17%
Average	25-31%	18-24%
Obese	32% +	25%+

The Harris-Benedict Formula for daily calorie needs

Basal Metabolic Rate = 655 + (9.6 x wt in kg)
+ (1.8 x ht in cm) – (4.7 x age in years)

1 inch = 2.54 cm

1 kg = 2.2 lbs.

Example:

- You are female
- You are 45 years old
- You are 5'2 tall (157.48)
- Your weigh 125 lbs (56.81 kg)

Your **BMR** = 655 + 545 + 283 - 211= **1272 calories per day**

Now that you know what your body needs just to function (i.e. for your eyes to blink, heart to beat, etc.), we need to factor in your activity level for the day. The following chart will help you estimate. If you are in question, always guess one level lower.

Activity Level Multiplier Description

- Sedentary BMR X 1.2 Little or no exercise, desk job
- Lightly Active BMR X 1.375 Light exercise or sports 3–5 days/week
- Moderately Active BMR X 1.55 Moderate exercise or sports 3–5 days/week
- Very Active BMR X 1.725 Hard exercise or sports 6–7 days/week
- Extremely Active BMR X 1.9 Hard daily exercise or sports and physical labor job or twice-a-day training (football camp, etc)
- Continuation of BMR example above:
- Your BMR is 1272 calories per day
- You have figured your activity level to be sedentary (little or no exercise)
- Your activity multiplier is 1.2
- Your total daily expenditure = 1.2 x 1272 = **1526 calories /day**

The Katch-McArdle Equation for daily calorie needs

The Harris-Benedict equation has separate formulas for men and women because men usually have larger bodies and more lean body mass. Since the Katch-McArdle formula accounts for LBM, this single formula applies equally to both men and women and it's the most accurate method for calculating your daily calorie needs.

BMR (men and women) = 370 + (21.6 X lean mass in kg)

Example:

You weigh 150 pounds (68 kg)
Your body fat percentage is 24% (36 pounds fat, 114 pounds lean)
Your lean mass is 114 pounds (51.8 kg)
Your BMR = 370 + (21.6 X 51.8) = **1489 calories**

To determine Total Daily Energy Expenditure from BMR, you simply multiply BMR by the activity factor, as shown in the following example:

Continuing with the previous example:

Your BMR is 1489
• Your activity level is moderately active
 (moderate workouts 3–4 times per week)
• Your activity factor is 1.55
• Your TDEE = 1.55 X 1821 = **2822 calories**

Activity Level Multiplier Description

• Sedentary BMR X 1.2 Little or no exercise, desk job
• Lightly Active BMR X 1.375 Light exercise or sports
 3–5 days/week
• Moderately Active BMR X 1.55 Moderate exercise or sports
 3–5 days/week
• Very Active BMR X 1.725 Hard exercise or sports
 6–7 days/week
• Extremely Active BMR X 1.9 Hard daily exercise or sports and
 physical labor job or twice-a-day training (football camp, etc)

Food Journal Helper

Breakfast	Time	Serving	Food Item	Protein(g)	Carbohydrates(g)	Fat(g)	Calories	Notes

Snack	Time	Serving	Food Item	Protein(g)	Carbohydrates(g)	Fat(g)	Calories	Notes

Lunch	Time	Serving	Food Item	Protein(g)	Carbohydrates(g)	Fat(g)	Calories	Notes

Snack	Time	Serving	Food Item	Protein(g)	Carbohydrates(g)	Fat(g)	Calories	Notes

Dinner	Time	Serving	Food Item	Protein(g)	Carbohydrates(g)	Fat(g)	Calories	Notes

Snack	Time	Serving	Food Item	Protein(g)	Carbohydrates(g)	Fat(g)	Calories	Notes
TOTALS								

Supportive Nutrition	Protein	Starchy Carb	Fibrous Carb	Calories
Breakfast				
Snack				
Lunch				
Snack				
Dinner				
Snack				

Resistance Training: Factor 2	LDS/Reps	LDS/Reps	LDS/Reps
	/	/	/
	/	/	/
	/	/	/
	/	/	/
	/	/	/
	/	/	/
	/	/	/
	/	/	/
Moderate Cardio: Factor 3	NOTES:		
Type:			
Minutes:			

My goal today:

My attitude today was:

Things I did today to be healthier:

Today, I Rewarded myself by:

I am most grateful for:

My biggest accomplishment today was:

My biggest setback today was:

Quick start calorie worksheet to reach your goal

1. Choose your goal
   a. Fat loss/muscle gain
   b. Weight gain

2. Figure out your daily calorie needs.
   a. Basal Metabolic Rate = 655 + (9.6 x wt in kg) +
   (1.8 x ht   in cm) – (4.7 x age in years)
   1 inch = 2.54 cm
   1 kg = 2.2 lbs.

Now that you know what your body needs just to function (i.e. for your eyes to blink, heart to beat, etc.), we need to factor in your activity level for the day. The following chart will help you estimate. If you are in question, always guess one level lower.

Activity Level Multiplier Description

Sedentary
BMR X 1.2 Little or no exercise, desk job

Lightly Active
BMR X 1.375 Light exercise or sports 3–5 days/week

Moderately Active
BMR X 1.55 Moderate exercise or sports 3–5 days/week

Very Active
BMR X 1.725 Hard exercise or sports 6–7 days/week

Extremely Active
BMR X 1.9 Hard daily exercise or sports and physical labor job or twice-a-day training (football camp, etc)

Continuation of BMR example above:

3. If goal is fat loss/muscle gain subtract 10-30% of daily expen diture to start losing fat. Never drop below 1200 calories with out medical supervision

a. If total daily expenditure =1526, then – (20%)305 calories = 1221 calories for fat loss

4. If goal is to add weight (fat free weight) add 10-30% to daily expenditure to gain.

5. Choose your workout :

a. Choose a strength work out and follow up with cardio in your zone *or*

b. Choose one of the recommended video sites which offer a good mix of cardio and strength all in one.

i. **Bodyrock.tv** is a free site

ii. **DailyBurn.com** offers a free 30 day trial

Our favorite recipes for any meal plan
Breaded Chicken Parmesan

Minutes to Prepare: 10
Minutes to Cook: 20
Number of Servings: 2

Ingredients

12 ounces white meat chicken
  (one double breast)
1 tbsp grated Parmesan cheese
1/4 cup Italian-style bread crumbs
1 tsp garlic powder
1 tbsp onions, dried
Crushed red peppers if desired
1 -2 tbsp olive oil

Nutritional Information

- Servings Per Recipe: 2
- Amount Per Serving
- Calories: 173.3
- Total Fat: 5.4 g
- Cholesterol: 38.5 mg
- Sodium: 323.4 mg
- Total Carbs: 13.6 g
- Dietary Fiber: 0.9 g
- Protein: 17.0 g

Directions

Cut the chicken breast horizontally (filet it) so you will end up with two thin pieces.

Rub each piece with olive oil.

Mix dry ingredients together and pat each piece with the crumb mixture until well covered.

Bake at 375*F for about 20 minutes.

Chicken Creole

Ingredients

Nonstick cooking spray as needed

4 medium chicken breast halves, skinned, boned, and cut into 1" strips

1 can (14 oz.) tomatoes, cut up
1 cup low-sodium chili sauce
1-1/2 cups green peppers, chopped (1 large)
1/2 cup celery, chopped
1/4 cup onion, chopped
2 cloves minced garlic
1 tablespoon fresh basil or 1 teaspoon dried
1 tablespoon fresh parsley or 1 teaspoon dried
1/4 teaspoon crushed red pepper
1/4 teaspoon salt

Directions

1. Spray a deep skillet with nonstick spray coating. Preheat pan over high heat.

2. Cook chicken in hot skillet, stirring, for 3-5 minutes, or until no longer pink. Reduce heat.

3. Add tomatoes and their juice, low-sodium chili sauce, green pepper, celery, onion, garlic, basil, parsley, crushed red pepper, and salt. Bring to boiling; reduce heat and simmer, covered, for 10 minutes.

Yield: 4 servings--

Serving Size: 1-1/2 cup.

Nutritional Information

• Amount Per Serving
• Calories: 255.4
• Total Fat: 4.5 g
• Cholesterol: 77.0 mg
• Sodium: 652.4 mg
• Total Carbs: 20.7 g
• Dietary Fiber: 4.3 g
• Protein: 33.3 g

Chicken Taco Soup

Ingredients

24 oz. chicken breast boneless skinless

2 cans of black beans – completely drained and rinsed

1 can of tomato sauce (8 oz)

1 can of diced tomatoes with oregano, basil and garlic (10 oz)

½ can Rotel tomatoes with green chiles

12 oz low sodium chicken broth

1 packet reduced sodium taco seasoning

Put all ingredients in crockpot and then put chicken in last. Cook for 5 hours on low. I scoop out the chicken after 5 hours and divide into 6 piles of 4oz each and put into containers. Then I scoop about ½ to 3/4 cup of beans and tomatoes into container and then pour the juice in to the consistency that you like (less liquid if you like thicker).

If you are not majorly concerned about getting 4oz of chicken pull chicken out after 5 hours and then shred and put back in the crock pot to cook for a couple hours.

Nutritional Information

Calories: 306

Protein: 35.8

Carbs: 36.8 (which is probably less because I drain the beans and didn't include dietary fiber)

Fat: 1.6

Two Bean Turkey Chili

1 lb. extra lean ground turkey
1 TBS dried minced onion
1 ½ tsp. garlic powder
4oz. can of green chilies (I only used 2 TBS.)
½ can reduced sodium black beans (Bush's)
   – RINSE AND DRAIN
½ can reduced sodium dark kidney beans (Bush's)
   – RINSE AND DRAIN
(1) 14oz can of organic diced tomatoes
seasoned with garlic/oregano – DO NOT DRAIN
2 tsp. splenda brown sugar
1 ½ tsp. chili powder
1 TBSP white vinegar
1 TBSP honey mustard
1 tsp. cumin
1/2 tsp. fine sea salt
Approximately 2 cups of chicken broth
and/or water to get to desired consistency.
1 ½ tsp. dried cilantro

Nutritional Information
• Amount Per Serving
• Calories: 282
• Protein: 40 g.
• Carbs: 26 g.
• Fat: 2.5 g.

Directions:

In a large skillet add meat and sprinkle with onions and garlic powder and cook until no longer pink (drain if needed).
Add the green chilies, beans, tomatoes, brown sugar and spices (everything except cilantro) and stir until combined.
Bring to a boil and reduce heat to simmer for about 10 minutes.
Add cilantro and serve hot.
May sprinkle veggie shreds or a light cheese on top.

Makes 4 servings (at approximately 5 oz per serving)

Sweet Potato Protein Pancake

150 grams sweet potato (baked and mashed)
1 scoop of whey protein powder (I use chocolate peanut butter)
3 egg whites
¼ tsp. baking soda
¼ tsp. baking powder
½ tsp. vanilla
½ tsp. nutmeg
1 tbsp. cinnamon
Dash of sea salt

Directions:

Heating skillet or griddle to medium heat, add just enough coconut oil to cover the surface/ bottom of skillet.

In a large bowl, mix all ingredients until smooth.

Drop about 1/4 to 1/3 cup size batter onto the skillet.

Cook 2-3 minutes. Flip and cook on other side 2-3 minutes.

Repeat for entire batch.

Top with sugar free syrup, cinnamon, agave, honey, almond butter, fruits, nuts, yogurt, whatever you prefer!! (Especially tasty with turkey bacon or sausage)

Nutritional Facts: (will vary somewhat on type of protein powder – mine is 24 g. protein, 5 carbs, 2.5 fat and 130 calories)

Serving Size: entire batch

Calories: 313
Carbs: 36.5g (dietary fiber 4.5g.)
Protein: 39g.
Fat: 2.5g.

Smoothies 300-400 calories each

Strawberry Blonde

- 10oz. milk or water
- ½ cup bananas
- ½ cup strawberries
- ¼ cup yogurt
- 1 scoop protein

The King

- 10oz. milk
- 1cup bananas
- 1scoop ice
- 2tbs. peanut butter
- 1scoop protein

Atomic Bomb

- 10oz. water or milk
- ¼ cup bananas
- ¼ cup blackberries
- ¼ cup strawberries
- ¼ cup blueberries
- ¼ cup yogurt
- 1 scoop protein

Be Berry

- 10oz. water or milk
- 2/3 cup raspberries
- 2/3 cup blackberries
- 2/3 cup blueberries
- ¼ cup yogurt
- 1 scoop of protein

Pinana

- 10oz. of water or milk
- 1 cup pineapples
- 1 cup bananas
- ¼ cup yogurt
- 1 scoop protein

Antioxidant Powerhouse

- 10oz. water or milk
- ¾ cup blueberries
- ¾ cup blackberries
- ½ cup spinach
- ¼ cup yogurt
- 1 scoop protein

PB&J

- 10oz. water or milk
- 2tbs. peanut butter
- 2/3 cup strawberries
- 2/3 cup blackberries
- 2/3 cup blueberries
- 1 scoop protein

Coco Banana

- 10oz. water or milk
- 1 cup banana
- 1 scoop chocolate protein
- 1 scoop ice

www.ingramcontent.com/pod-product-compliance
Lightning Source LLC
Chambersburg PA
CBHW050126280326
41933CB00010B/1273